Super Body, Super Brain

SUPER BODY, SUPER BRAIN

The Workout That Does It All

Michael Gonzalez-Wallace

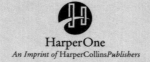

HarperOne
An Imprint of HarperCollinsPublishers

HarperOne

SUPER BODY, SUPER BRAIN: *The Workout That Does It All*. Copyright © 2010 by Michael Gonzalez-Wallace. All rights reserved. Printed in the United States of America. No part of this book may be used or reproduced in any manner whatsoever without written permission except in the case of brief quotations embodied in critical articles and reviews. For information, address HarperCollins Publishers, 10 East 53rd Street, New York, NY 10022.

HarperCollins books may be purchased for educational, business, or sales promotional use. For information, please write: Special Markets Department, HarperCollins Publishers, 10 East 53rd Street, New York, NY 10022.

HarperCollins website: http://www.harpercollins.com
HarperCollins®, ★®, and HarperOne™ are trademarks of HarperCollins Publishers

FIRST EDITION
Designed by Chris Rhoads
Photography by Keith Barraclough

Library of Congress Cataloging-in-Publication Data is available upon request.

ISBN 978–0–06–194527–4

10 11 12 13 14   RRD (H) 9 8 7 6 5 4 3 2 1

To my family, my clients,
and Dr. John Martin

SUPER BODY

contents

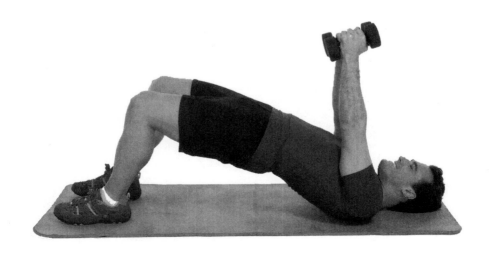

SUPER BRAIN

PART TWO
Exercises

PART THREE
Eating Plan

Foreword

As an neurobiologist, I've always been enthralled by how the brain orchestrates movement—how a pitcher can throw a ball and hit his mark or how a ballerina commands an incredible leap through the air. So it is easy to understand why I find Michael Gonzalez-Wallace's program so fascinating. Simply put, Michael has created a deceptively easy way to make the most of how our brain's motor circuits work (all while getting a great workout, no less!). Motor circuits are the networks of nerve cell connections that enable us to perform the full range of our everyday movements, like reaching for a cup of coffee or tying a knot. Even the act of inserting a key into a lock uses many brain regions, so you can imagine that the simple yet challenging movements you will learn to perform in *Super Body, Super Brain* drive up brain activity enormously. And when a brain region is more active, it makes new connections so it can perform its job better, faster, and more efficiently.

Long-standing scientific observation has already shown that aerobic exercise benefits cognitive functions in children and adults. Michael's program is not only highly aerobic, but cognitive as well, in that it requires the participant to learn and perform complex movements. The *Super Body, Super Brain* program is a particularly efficient way to improve brain functions as it makes us more agile and fit.

Even simple, everyday actions are perceived by the brain as quite complicated. But the kinds of movements Michael teaches demand even more of our motor circuits. All of our voluntary movements have a goal, and our brain plans the movement ahead of time—a sort of mental rehearsal. We may have only one chance to complete a movement, so we want our movements to succeed. As each action unfolds, the brain makes on-the-fly corrections to ensure that it is successful. Not surprisingly, when we make a relatively automatic or well-practiced movement—think about how many steps we take throughout the day or keys we type—our brain can more easily plan the movement. When we learn to make complex movements, though, our brain is forced to work harder. Michael's program is rich in movements that are new and not practiced, which require us to coordinate our bodies in ways that are very different from what we are accustomed to. This is much like reading a challenging novel. When we do, we must not only think about the meaning of individual words, and how the author combines the words into phrases with complex meanings, but we also might create a mental image of the story's actions. But unlike reading a difficult passage in a book—where we can take our time and re-read it, if necessary—we almost always have to perform these complex movements quickly. Picture a waiter bringing a bowl of soup to a table: one small mistake can snowball into a much bigger one that the customer will not appreciate! From one second to the next, the waiter's brain must adjust his balance and arm position, while he navigates tables, chairs, and people. Those complex tasks, like the exercises in this book, are every bit as demanding as reading and reasoning.

As various brain regions are recruited during *Super Body, Super Brain*'s exercise sequences, they become more active and, importantly, form new connections. This is simply the basic functioning of the brain. It is never static. When one part of the brain is more active, it changes both its internal connections and its connections with other parts of the brain. Existing connections are made stronger. Brand-new connections are made. Unused and unnecessary connections are eliminated. These modified connections are produced by many different kinds of biological mechanisms. One kind requires proteins that are called trophic factors. These proteins help to strengthen existing connections and form new connections. Active neurons produce these factors that help attract new connections. Withholding trophic factors can lead to eliminating unused connections. We think that the particular ways neurons become active during performance of a task will influence how proteins that are important in forming connections are made and used.

Not only do the kinds of movements in *Super Body, Super Brain* form new connections in the brain, they form them in regions that have diverse functions, like the cerebral cortex, cerebellum, basal ganglia, and hippocampus. That's particularly important, because many parts of these regions are not primarily associated with movement. They're actually better known for their roles in cognition, emotions, and memory. But as you perform movements that involve combinations of arm and leg movements, your brain has to multitask—as it does, it builds new connections between these crucial parts of the brain.

And those benefits don't end when your workout does. Because you're conditioning your brain to perform a complex task, not just making your muscles stronger, you'll begin to improve other brain functions, like paying attention and thinking. Michael's exercises require concentration, attention, and thinking, not just coordination, balance, and good timing. Brain imaging studies show that some of the same brain regions that become active during challenging movements, like the cerebellum and basal ganglia, also become active when we speak, read, and reason. Research suggests that it may not matter so much how we strengthen neural circuits. What is more important is *that* we strengthen them. And once made stronger—by performing Michael's exercise program, for example—those stronger neural circuits help us in countless other ways.

The *Super Body, Super Brain* program makes the brain work overtime—not just the parts that control our muscles and joints, but parts that participate in a wide range of everyday tasks. Moreover, this program is not static. Once we get it right, we move on to the next more difficult level, which helps keep our brain regions active. But let's not forget one last thing: the exercises in *Super Body, Super Brain* also make us fit! There is an exquisite synergy between the aerobic benefits of these lively and challenging movements, the way they activate the brain, and the biological benefits you'll see as a result of your increasingly stimulated brain circuits. *Super Body, Super Brain* adds up to be an excellent cognitive workout masquerading as a smart, efficient way to condition your body. Give it a try, and see for yourself how our bodies and our brains work together in a rich and productive collaboration. *Super Body, Super Brain* is one workout that this neuroscientist wholeheartedly endorses!

John H. Martin, Ph.D.

It is exercise alone that lifts the spirits,
and keeps the mind in vigor.

—CICERO

Introduction

Who doesn't want to get smarter?

Brain fitness is big business. Bookstores and libraries have shelves lined with crossword-puzzle books, memory teasers, books of sudoku, DVDs, software games—you name it—all promising to increase your cognitive powers for optimal brain functioning. But the one thing nearly all of these books and products have in common is this: they ignore *movement*.

And what part of your body controls movement—along with balance, coordination, posture, and decisions about how and when to execute any movement?

Your *brain,* of course.

Super Body, Super Brain is an incredibly effective and efficient progressive exercise program—the first of its kind. By spending a mere ten minutes a day at home, without any equipment other than a few hand weights, you will burn calories, improve your balance and coordination, make your muscles and cardiovascular system stronger without impacting your joints, and improve your learning power and concentration at the same time. (You'll be doing over six hundred movements in less than ten minutes!) Add another ten to twenty minutes, and you will maximize your results. In fact, I'll show you how breaking up your exercise time into ten-minute segments not only is as productive as doing one longer session, but makes finding the time to exercise particularly easy no matter how busy you are.

In this book I incorporate the latest research in neuroscience, fitness, and nutrition. You'll notice that the Super Body, Super Brain movements are deceptively simple. Conventional (boring) exercises (like a plain old biceps curl) use limited areas of the brain. But whenever you do one of my exercises, you'll activate many more areas of your brain: the cerebellum, your brain's inner computer, responsible for balance, coordination, intentional and skilled movement, muscle timing, and speech; the basal ganglia, the part of the brain involved with motor-coordinated movements; the motor cortex; the hippocampus, in charge of learning new movements; and the frontal lobes, which are responsible for higher thinking and decision making.

So even though your brain is not a muscle, you can use your muscles to boost your brainpower. The principle is clear: when you use several muscles at once, you need to think about what you're doing. Sounds like a breeze, right? Actually, this simple thought process is what gives your brain a jolt of pure power.

And here's the reason: not every movement is created equal. Each Super Body, Super Brain exercise may seem easy to perform, but the crucial element is that *your brain perceives the exercises as challenging.*

If you don't believe me, close your eyes, and then raise one leg and hold it steady for ten seconds while clapping. It's surprisingly tough to do. That's because when you close your eyes, you literally see with your brain (which I'll discuss in chapter 1). And your brain, being challenged with such a surprising task, isn't quite up to it yet. But after only a very few weeks of practice, you'll be able to close your eyes and do an amazing variety of movements you never thought you could.

That's because Super Body, Super Brain gives you the best of both worlds: exercises demanding balance, coordination, and con-

centration for a superior brain workout, combined with aerobic, strength-training moves that rev up your metabolism and make your muscles lean and strong.

Do these Super Body, Super Brain exercises regularly, and in less than a month you will:

• **Lose weight and reduce your body fat.** When you use strength training and the constant motion of the Super Body, Super Brain exercises, you will reduce stored fat, increase lean muscle, and thus automatically increase your metabolism. And if you make changes to your diet (covered in chapter 13) at the same time, you will see results even more quickly.

• **Strengthen all your core muscles as well as tone the muscles in your upper and lower body.** Each workout engages so many different muscle groups that you'll be working them all simultaneously and efficiently.

• **Strengthen your heart and lungs and improve your endurance.** These exercises are aerobic, so they burn as many calories as running does for the average person—but without any high-impact stress on your joints. Using low weights and high repetitions will deliver a simultaneous strength-training and aerobic workout.

• **Improve your balance and coordination.** Think about dance, and coordination comes to mind; think about yoga, and you'll focus on balance. Balance and coordination need to be working simultaneously. With Super Body, Super Brain, you'll start with a coordinated movement, and your intention is to move your body into a challenging, balanced position. This is what makes my program so unique: this synced-up, harmonious integration of balance and coordination will stimulate both brain and body. It is integral to every circuit in this book.

I also want to avoid one of the causes of injuries to dancers. The constant repetition and muscle tension that make dancers strong and fluid can also involve a tremendous amount of rotation, which puts a huge amount of stress on joints and soft tissues.

• **Transform your posture and become more flexible.** One of the best elements of Super Body, Super Brain is that there is only one way to do the movements—the correct way! Because you need to concentrate so powerfully on executing each movement, you must be perfectly aligned. So you'll never have to worry that you're expending time, energy, and hard work and not getting the desired results!

• **Improve your alertness and lessen fatigue.** Exercising at a moderate intensity lessens fatigue, as it helps regulate neurotransmitter levels, which is why regular exercisers have more energy and sleep better than those who are sedentary.

• **Become more mentally sharp, with improved memory capability.** Whenever you move, your brain snaps into action in a remarkably choreographed sequence of signals from the nerve cells to the muscles and back again. The more challenging your movements, the more different areas of your brain will be stimulated and strengthened.

But your body is also a marvel of efficiency, so as it gets used to exercise routines, it tends to minimize its energy input. If you follow my program and constantly switch it up, as I show you how to do, you'll trick your body into producing maximum results with minimal difficulty! You'll burn a lot more calories. And you'll never get bored, since how you're moving always challenges your brain in a deceptively simple way.

• **Improve your mood.** Allowing your brain to guide you through these exercises not only will keep it stimulated and sharp but can affect your *feelings* and mood as well. The perceived novelty of learning new movements excites several neurotransmitters (particularly dopamine, serotonin, and endorphins) in your brain, which affect your sense of well-being and are crucial for modulating anxiety and depression.

As child psychiatrist and member of my advisory board Dr. Gregory Lombardo explained to me, "There's a transformation. What we are talking about are changes in the way thoughts and feelings operate, as well as how the muscles and the cerebellum are stimulated."

• **Do a maximum workout in minimal space and in minimal time.** Although I hope that everyone will try to do at least twenty to thirty minutes of Super Body, Super Brain exercises several times a week, you will see results if you do as little as ten minutes of exercises a day.

Plus, you need only a very small space, and can do your circuits just about anywhere—at home, at the office, in a hotel room, at the beach; you can even do some of the movements at a bus stop or while waiting for an elevator. You can also do this workout with your family, especially your children; your friends; or your colleagues at work during a break. Not only is the routine quick, but it costs almost nothing, aside from the cost of hand weights. (And you can even start with soup cans!)

Crunching More Than Numbers

I think I can safely say that I'm one of the few personal trainers in New York City who used to be an investment banker. Banking was a career that I loved, but as a former competitive athlete who'd been involved in sports for over two decades, I realized that my fascination with human performance was even more enticing. I decided to keep the best aspects of finance (constant mental stimulation, creative and progressively challenging strategies, the desire and need to see tangible results) and apply them to my passion for fitness, and I became certified as a personal trainer. Early in my newfound career, I was building a client base by working in gyms in New York City. I was thrilled when my first private client hired me for a session in her home . . . until I walked in the door. Not only were her kids running around, competing for Mom's attention, but I realized that I didn't have the variety of offerings of a gym, where I could take clients to different exercise machines. What was I going to do? I had to get creative.

And not just with her—with all of my growing number of private clients. Most of them were brilliantly successful, too busy with work and family to go to the gym. They bluntly stated that they hated to work out even though they knew they had to do it, and they were willing to give me precisely two sessions a week in which I had to whip them into shape. Not only did they expect an aerobic, heart-pumping, calorie-burning workout, but they expected the exercises to be gentle on their joints while firming and toning their muscles—with only exercise mats, a pair of hand weights, a whole lot of expectations, and me. Wow!

And because these were incredibly smart people at the top of their game, used to tough daily challenges, they brought the same can-do, don't-let-me-down-or-else attitude to their workouts. I had to get them physically fit while keeping them with me mentally.

I had to come up with a powerful, effective fitness program that produced maximum results in minimal time, and I had to do it fast. What were all the variables I needed to consider?

I thought back to my economics classes, where I'd learned how to forecast and correlate independent variables. For instance, inflation is dependent on different variables, such as how much money is invested or how much disposable income people have to spend, among others. And then I had one of those incredibly invigorating *Eureka!* moments when I realized I could apply the same kind of econometric forecasting model to a structured, progressive exercise program. Combining these variables into one seamless, flowing whole would give me an absolutely comprehensive circuit.

First, there were the elements of balance and coordination—those things that keep us from walking like robots!

Next, it had to be something dynamic, yet gentle enough not to put any stress or impact on aging joints. I had already noticed how having my clients multitask by doing strength-training movements increased their heart rate. The benefits of strength training have been extensively studied: as you gain muscle and lose fat, you rev up your metabolism (since muscles burn calories faster than fat); your heart is strengthened and your blood pressure decreases; your blood sugar, insulin, and cholesterol levels stabilize; and strong muscles help with the alignment and mobility of your joints.

So I asked a few eager client volunteers to wear a heart-rate monitor so we could test different exercise combinations to discover which specific movements either raised or lowered their heart rate. This allowed me to create the most powerful *flow* of specific movements.

It had to be super-efficient, a workout that could be done anywhere, by anyone no matter what their size or shape or level of athletic ability, in as little time as possible.

It had to be a workout that would be progressive, and it had to be infinitely customizable so it would keep my clients' interest even as their skill level improved.

And most of all, it had to be a workout that really worked, that would easily become part of anyone's daily routine so they would be able to do it for a lifetime.

At that point, I must confess, I wasn't yet thinking about brainpower—I was thinking only about keeping my clients happy so they wouldn't fire me! I spent the next few weeks crafting a routine with constant repetition of the superpotent strength-training movements. My clients were thrilled when their bodies quickly began to transform and the pounds melted away, but *I* still wasn't satisfied with my sessions.

One day when I was training a male client in his sumptuous apartment, I realized that he had mentally checked out. Oh sure, he was still doing his biceps curls, but I could tell that his thoughts were wandering. How was I going to motivate this man who was very successful, driven, not used to being told what to do—and about to fire me?

Then I had a flash, a memory from my basketball days. How did I break down the movement to shoot a basket? First I'd bend my knees; then I'd simultaneously raise my heels up only a few inches while lifting up my arms, aiming for the basket. That motion demanded perfect balance, coordination, strength, precision, and reflexes—or I'd miss by a mile.

What I'd forgotten about was *intent*—the mind-set and goal of getting the ball into the basket. Intent is, literally, all in your head. It demands perfect focus and clarity. It forces your brain to work, and work hard. Just as you select your words with intent before you speak or write, or as you use intent to make your daily decisions, you can use intent to move your muscles. Tell yourself how you need to move, and your brain will click into action, boosted with its own power to instantly plan and execute your intended movements.

Why not try something similar with this bored client? Why not incorporate balance, coordination, precision, and intent into the strength-training routine he was grumbling about? If I did, what would happen?

"OK, now do that shoulder raise with a calf raise at the same time," I told him. Grudgingly, he started doing the movement, and his face suddenly changed. The boredom evaporated. He had to think—*really* think—about what he was doing.

"Now do a squat-plié, and when you're starting to come up, raise your arms at the same time," I said, deliberately switching up the timing, too.

He tried to do this combination of two movements he'd done separately many times before, then shook his head. "Walk me through it," he said. He was engaged. He was focused. Very soon, he was dripping with sweat.

"What just happened?" he asked when the session was over. "That was the best workout *ever*."

What happened was that I'd forced him to multitask as if he'd been directing a board meeting at work, to engage not only his muscles but his brain. He'd unwittingly been so challenged and had to think so intently about not toppling over that he'd had to give his best without knowing it. Adding the mental component had suddenly transformed the same old workout into something altogether extraordinary.

My mind was racing as I walked home. Why had that session been so incredible? Oh, *of course:* it was the power of concentration in action. My client had been forced to turn off the autopilot I was seeing on the faces of the bored and tuned-out runners who passed me by.

I'd totally overlooked the most important element of any workout. Not just muscles, or breathing, or weights, or speed—but the *brain*. By combining balance, coordination, and intent with potent strength training, I'd literally seen how you *can* train your brain and your muscles at the same time!

I guess you could say Super Body, Super Brain was born in the living rooms of my clients. This amazing journey has taken me from Park Avenue apartments to the offices of some of the world's top neuro-scientists, brain researchers, physiologists, and psychiatrists, and, now, into the pages of this book.

Waking Up the Brain: The Further Evolution of Super Body, Super Brain

As I thought more about the connection between muscle power and brainpower, I began to notice startling differences in my clients. Those who were young, from age thirteen up to about age forty, were ecstatic at seeing how quickly they were developing long, lean, well-defined muscles all over their body as well as powerful core strength that rid of them of the flabby bellies and butts that had driven them crazy for years. Plus, they went from looking at me blankly when I told them how to move to memorizing and flawlessly repeating complicated sequences within a scant few weeks of their introduction.

My older clients, in the forty-five- to seventy-five-year-old age bracket, were altogether different. At first, most of them were out of shape and moved hesitantly. If I said, "Raise your right arm and your left leg at the same time," they needed several long seconds to process, visualize, and execute the move—after asking me to show them first. They also had problems doing simultaneous balance and coordination movements without jerking or stopping.

But after several weeks of constant struggle, these clients' movements suddenly became smooth, strong, and speedy—as if switching from a dial-up modem to high-speed broadband. We were all elated, particularly as these changes were especially noticeable in my clients over sixty. What had triggered such an amazing transformation?

It wasn't just stronger muscles. Something had woken up in their brains.

At this point, I became a man obsessed, researching everything I could find about the brain. In my neuroanatomy textbooks, I learned that 50 percent of all neurons (nerve cells) are found in 10 percent of brain mass—in the cerebellum—and that this 10 percent is responsible for balance and coordination, muscle timing, and postural alignment as well as cognitive functions like speech and problem solving.

It was another one of those *Eureka!* moments. I'd instinctively created an exercise system that was stimulating the most potent part of the brain.

In my research, I learned that the brain could be rewired after learning specific movements. I also found that instead of doing traditional research—comparing results from animals that exercise to those that don't—scientists were comparing animals that exercised but that did so in different ways. They discovered that animals whose brains were challenged during exercise not only increased brain activity but actually got smarter. Applying those same brain-challenging principles to the exercises I'd already created would be absolutely ideal, wouldn't it?

And then I thought, Why not take it further, and have this program incorporate sets of structured, progressive exercises that would *always* lead to quantifiable results, much as a composer would build a symphony by layering one musical line atop another? This exercise system would *always* get the best out of bodies and brains at the same time.

At this stage, I needed more—I needed tangible explanations of *how* and *why* from neuroscientists to confirm my theories. How was I going to find these experts?

Starbucks Changed My Life

Sitting with some research papers in a Starbucks in early 2006, I noticed a lovely young woman at the next table, reading a neurology textbook. (What can I say? I'm a Spaniard, after all!) We started talking, and when she told me she was a first-year medical student at Columbia University, I eagerly told her what I was working on.

"Well," she said, showing me a book I had already read, *Neuroanatomy: Text and Atlas,* "why don't you contact the guy who wrote this? This is the standard textbook for all first-year medical students. His name is John Martin, and he's one of my professors. He teaches clinical neurobiology and behavior." Then she wrote down his e-mail address on a napkin as I silently thanked my flirtation genes.

I still can't believe how fortuitous that chance meeting was: I soon found out that Dr. Martin is an expert on the body's motor system and on linking the connections between the brain and movement. Perfect!

So I e-mailed him, asking for advice, and was thrilled when he wrote me right back to set up a meeting. Luckily, we hit it off right away—probably because my nerves got the most of me and I blurted out, "John, I just want to know if I'm crazy or not! Am I on the right track?"

Indeed I was. John was amazed that someone with only a layman's knowledge of neuroscience had already invented a circuit with unique movements that required intense brain activity—the kind likely to create reserves of new neurons as well as strengthen preexisting connections in the brain's action systems. He confirmed that it is possible to challenge muscles by using no-impact exercises that are safe for everyone to do, while maximizing brain activity at the same time. Your brain *can* keep learning no matter how old you are—but *only* if you challenge it and are consistent with these challenges, doing the same sort of mental and physical exercises on a regular basis. "Perhaps, the more you need to think during a complex movement, the more you recruit connections in the cognitive systems of the brain," he told me. "If you can get people to do these movements before they really start slowing down, you might be able to help decelerate their problems with balance and coordination, and potentially slow down brain loss or deterioration."

As we continued to meet, John encouraged me to ratchet the program up to another level. "You could help a lot of people with this program, since motor skills are essential if we want to function well. Not only do your exercises require coordination, but initiating the movements and being able to stabilize them requires intense brain and muscle function," he said, then smiled. "It's easier to read Ian Fleming than James Joyce, you know," he added. "You're turning into the James Joyce of exercise!"

"The Workout That Does It All"

I didn't realize how hungry people were for an efficient, multitasking workout until an article about the early phase of Super Body, Super Brain, entitled "The Workout That Does It All," appeared in *O, The Oprah Magazine* in March 2006.

Although there were only four exercises in that short article, my e-mail in-box soon overflowed, with nearly everyone telling me that they didn't like to go to the gym yet were desperate to exercise. Did I have more exercises for them? Could I explain how exercise could stimulate brain activity and cognitive powers to help them get smarter and stronger at the same time?

Indeed I could. So I've spent the last few years consulting dozens more neuroscientists, neurokinesiologists, physicians, psychiatrists, and brain researchers from all over the world. I kept working until I knew that my system was infallible. I was able to

meld brain science with what I saw every day with my clients—that Super Body, Super Brain exercises *do* have an effect on brainpower. And now you can do them, too.

How to Use This Book

In part 1, you'll learn the basics behind the brain–muscle connection, seeing how exercise and learning new movements can literally rewire and stimulate our brains.

Part 2 covers the exercise circuits. Chapter 5 gives you all the basics, and chapters 6 through 9 cover the four primary levels, with exercises that you'll master over a four-week period. These exercises become progressively more challenging.

Once you've mastered them, chapter 10 will show you how to use the different levels in a unique, progressive sequence that will always keep you challenged. Finally, you'll come to the Master Circuit for the ultimate workout.

Several more chapters will spotlight the power of Super Body, Super Brain for all readers: chapter 11 will show you the power of walking, which will add an entirely new element of strength and coordination to your workouts. Chapter 12 contains unique exercise routines for the entire family, as well as for seniors who may want a gentler introduction to exercise.

In part 3, chapter 13 gives you sensational new information about the best brain foods as well as a diet plan with delectable, supernutritious recipes. Good nutrition is a huge and often overlooked factor when tackling brain function, especially for those who concentrate solely on weight loss. Based in the latest research, I've devised a powerful program with the help of a top nutritionist, Olinka Podany.

I want to make personal training accessible to everyone, and I hope that you will consider this book as the equivalent of my private training sessions. So, for example, the name of each exercise in part 2 is the exact same verbal command that I give to my clients. Consider these instructions the equivalent of me being in the room, right there with you, cheering you on. Follow the plan, and get ready to see remarkable changes in a matter of weeks.

Most of all, I want you to have the same *Eureka!* moment I had when I realized that the untapped power of the brain could transform a boring old exercise routine into something that can change your body and your thinking.

I want you to believe that the Super Body, Super Brain philosophy is not just about adding movement into your life so that you can lose weight or tone up your muscles. I've always been puzzled as to why anyone would start an exercise regimen simply to lose a few extra pounds in the short term when the truly important long-term issue is their *health*.

I know that many people quit their training because they're not getting the results they think they want. But that's a huge mistake, because you need to believe in yourself and in the vitally important task that you are about to undertake once you realize that training is not about fitting into a new dress but about building a strong and resilient body and a strong and powerful brain. It is about extending your life and creating a confident, smart, and unstoppable you.

Making the exercises in this book a regular part of your life is like making the choice between driving a beat-up old jalopy and a turbocharged racecar. Both will get you to your destination, but only one will do so with maximum power.

And believe me when I tell you that you already possess the best turbocharged racecar on the market: your very own brain. The power is yours! Once you start doing the Super Body, Super Brain exercises, you can build and turbocharge your neurons, giving you the best-functioning brain you can possibly have—for life.

PART ONE

SUPER BODY, SUPER BRAIN

The Basics Behind the Brain–Muscle Connection

1

The softening of the body involves a serious weakening of the mind.

—SOCRATES

The Brain–Muscle Connection

One of the more annoying math teachers I had in high school was fond of taunting his students by saying, "Get it through your thick skulls now, while you're young, or you'll never get it at all!"

Well, I am thrilled to report that this boring old fuddy-duddy was wrong—because what neuroscientists have learned in the last decade has upended long-held assumptions about brain function. Instead of reaching its full capacity when you're too young to appreciate it and then beginning an inexorable decline down the slippery slope to senility, your amazing brain is astonishingly dynamic and adaptable. Even better, it continues to grow and form new connections based on all your experiences throughout your entire life: it constantly rewires itself in a process known as *neuroplasticity*.

And it's never too late to start. I've seen remarkable improvement in many people who are in their seventies and eighties, even if they're newcomers to exercise. As soon as you start learning my coordination patterns, you'll create more, stronger, and more powerful synapses (the spaces between the neurons in your brain) and will allow your brain to become and stay more resilient. What you'll have is a better brain–muscle connection.

How do you do that? One of the best ways to stimulate the growth of new neural connections is with the element of *surprise*.

Surprise your brain when you force it to think and concentrate in a powerful new way with *movement,* and you'll create new neural pathways, improve your neuromuscular coordination, and stop forgetting where you put the keys. And when you surprise your muscles with new exercise patterns at the same time, they'll become and stay long, lean, toned, and strong.

The element of surprise is also a perfect way to keep your brain running at peak efficiency. Think of how you feel when you're driving to work on a route you've taken a thousand times before. It's awfully easy to tune out, isn't it? But if you're driving a different route for the first time, your brain is surprised by all this new information. Your senses are on high alert. Your brain is concentrating, multitasking, focusing, and making instant decisions so you can arrive at your destination.

But if you start driving on this new route without incident every day, you'll soon tune out again. That's because your brain is not just clever; it's hyperefficient. It just loves to shut off unused and unneeded circuits to conserve energy. Adding the element of surprise is what keeps it tuned up.

The same thing happens when you exercise. If the kind of *movement* you do is based on the element of surprise in an ever-changing, progressively challenging circuit, your brain can't shut down. The information it receives whenever you do the Super Body, Super Brain exercises doesn't require just any plain old kind of concentration, but a very specific type of cognitive processing that instantaneously sends information in new ways, to all parts of your brain—some of which you may not even know you're using. Even better, it processes the sensory feedback from your muscles and joints to your brain, too. Being able to quickly take in and respond to this information is what pushes your brain into hyperdrive and gives it a challenging and satisfying workout. This can help extend your brain's potential to keep working at full speed throughout your entire life.

So let's take a look at how you can boost your brainpower with movement.

Plug It In and Get Supercharged: Rewire Your Brain with Movement

When I started researching brain function, one of the first books I picked up was John Ratey's *A User's Guide to the Brain.* Deep in the reading one day, I came across three momentous sentences: "What makes us move is also what makes us think," Dr. Ratey wrote. "Our physical movements can directly influence our ability to learn, think, and remember. Evidence is mounting that each person's capacity to master new and remember old information is improved by biological changes in the brain brought on by physical activity."

My jaw dropped. He'd put words to what I'd already noticed, because my private clients kept telling me how much more *clar-*

ity they had with their thinking, whether at work or at home, after doing the Super Body, Super Brain exercises. Not only that, but they relished the challenges of every workout, mastering each new level and preparing for the next one. The adrenaline rush was hitting not just their muscles but their brains!

These clients were living proof that exercise can truly ignite our brainpower, and that challenging exercises make us think and dig deep to find the best within ourselves.

"Use It or Lose It" Isn't Just for Muscles: It's What Neuroplasticity Does in Your Brain

"Use it or lose it" is a phrase you hear a lot, whether in the gym or the research lab. If you don't use your muscles, they wither in atrophy. And if you don't use your brain, it can wither in its own way, too. Without constant stimulation, it just can't stay sharp.

Anytime you learn anything—mental or physical, complicated or ludicrously simple—you create new synapses as well as strengthen preexisting synapses in your brain through a process called *neuroplasticity*. This kind of plasticity has nothing to do with plastic food wrap or storage containers and everything to do with your brain as "plastic" in the sense of being highly adaptable to stimulus and change. Your brain is literally set up so you can keep on learning from day one to the end of your days.

But it's all too easy to misperceive neuroplasticity as something that's just about

cognitive ability or intellectual function, believing that you can keep your brain in peak shape only through the use of words or numbers—by doing crossword puzzles or sudoku or by learning a new language. Doing so leaves out the vital importance of *movement* in brain stimulation.

How movement can affect brain function was proven in a well-known study by a neuroscientist, William Greenough, and others in 1991. In this study, rats that exercised in enriched environments were found to have a greater number of synaptic connections than rats that just sat around eating in their cages all day. The amount of movement that the mobile rats had while running on a wheel made their brains grow stronger and smarter.

Fortunately, the same thing happens in our brains, as I discussed with Dr. Wendy Suzuki, associate professor of neural science and psychology at New York University. Learning new movements not only increases the size of your neurons and the number of synapses in your brain's motor cortex and cerebellum and other areas in the brain, but also creates new neural connections as the neurons in one area of the brain communicate with neurons in other parts of the brain. (Neuroscientists call this *integration and projection*.)

Even better, the more your brain perceives movements as complicated, even when *you* might not think they are, the more brain activity is stimulated. I made use of this phenomenon in structuring the progressive element in the Super Body,

Super Brain exercises, so that you can reap the benefits every time you do a circuit.

Neurogenesis: Keep on Churning Out New Neurons

Whenever you learn something new or do something new, certain areas of the brain light up and create new neurons as if you'd just plugged in the cerebral Christmas tree—what's called *neurogenesis*. Not only that, but these new neurons will function for much longer if you are exercising; if you're sedentary, existing neurons begin to naturally degenerate.

Neurogenesis primarily takes place in two different areas of the brain. The first is in the olfactory bulb, which helps you smell, among other functions. This is likely a leftover from early human days when a keen sense of smell could mean the dif-ference between catching your dinner or starving to death.

The other is the dentate gyrus of the hippocampus, important for learning and forming new memories. This is one of the areas with the highest neurogenesis rates. Furthermore, according to a study done by Scott A. Small, M.D., at Columbia University, a three-month aerobic exercise program consistently brought more blood flow to the hippocampus, helping it function better. Another study, headed by Dr. Art Kramer at the University of Illinois, showed how aerobic exercise brought measurably improved blood volume to the hippocampus as well as the frontal cortex and temporal cortex of older adults' brains. (For more on the hippocampus, see page 24.)

This is particularly pertinent for Super Body, Super Brain, because the hippocam-

rory's story

"I needed to have several brain surgeries in 2006 and developed epilepsy in 2007. During one of the surgeries, I had a stroke. My balance and gait were all out of whack and I had a lot of trouble moving anywhere without falling over, but the physical therapy I had at several different medical centers in New York City wasn't helping me as much as I'd hoped.

"Michael's training was a lot different. After only a few sessions, my balance and my gait were a lot better. I felt this was due to his exercises working my brain as well as my muscles. He explained to me that our brains can keep growing and changing, even after an injury, which spurred me on to work even harder at getting my strength back."

pus helps you learn new things and retain this new information. And what you learn can be either word-based (like Scrabble skills) or physical (like new exercises). According to Dr. John Martin, this may be similar to creating a cognitive reserve by learning a new language later in life, or learning to play a musical instrument. The exercises likely drive more neural activity in more parts of the brain, and this can strengthen neural connections in the action systems of the brain.

These findings were noted in the research of Dr. Scott Small at Columbia University, and by Henrietta Van Praag at the National Institutes of Health as reported in the *Journal of Neurosciences* in 2005 and supported by several other studies.

Neuroscientists are deep on the trail of trying to discover whether neurogenesis can also take place regularly in other areas of the brain, particularly the cerebellum. One Italian study by neuroscientist Luca Bonfanti at the University of Turin did find evidence of neurogenesis in the hippocampus *and* cerebellum of rabbits. This has enormously positive implications—particularly that new stimulation through exercise and specific movements could create new neurons all over the brain.

But this is all cutting-edge stuff, since neurogenesis is still such a new concept for brain researchers. We do know that, as with other cells in the body, you lose neurons and then regain them in an endless cycle of cell death and birth. Obviously, you want to minimize the losses

and maximize the gains, but there are other implications to consider. Are all new neurons good cells, for example? We just don't know yet.

The key until we better understand more from this growing area of research is to keep stimulating the brain in such a way that it will be forced not only to create new neurons but to create more, and stronger, synapses connecting all these new neurons to other preexisting and new neurons. Which is precisely what the exercises of Super Body, Super Brain do: the more complex connections are created in the brain through the stimulation of new movement, the more other areas in the brain become involved. This leads to an endless cycle of new neural connections. You can challenge these neurons with specific movements the same way you challenge them with cognitive tests, leading to lasting new connections between your brain and your muscles.

I saw this every day when I was devising this program. My clients and I were always thrilled when they learned and remembered the sequence of movements amazingly quickly. Soon, all I had to do was give them a shorthand command (such as, "Leg straight behind biceps curl"), and they would know what to do without having to visualize it. It was as if their brains were literally creating a new code to match the movements.

Believe me, your brain will create the exact same code after you've done these exercises only a handful of times. You'll be able to learn and remember every single exercise in the sequence in less than a week!

Your Brain Can Use Muscles Like Words to Supercharge Itself to the Next Level

Whenever you do the Super Body, Super Brain exercises, with their precise and perfectly structured elements of balance and coordination, many different areas of your brain instantly respond. But they don't respond merely by one area lighting up in response and then another; instead, many different areas are stimulated and constantly send out signals to each other.

Picture all these different parts of the brain as one enormous interconnected circuit sending off information as one flawlessly integrated whole. It's an endlessly complicated and intricately structured web where, ideally, all the interconnective strands are as strong and supple as possible—so that all the neurons and synapses work in an endlessly flowing stream as well as they possibly can.

How does this happen? Well, the main reason is that your brain is a truly unique marvel. It's one of the most complex organs in your body, weighing about three pounds. This accounts for only 2 percent of the average person's body weight, but the brain consumes approximately 20 percent of the body's blood supply.

The average brain contains about one hundred billion neurons. Unlike the rest of the cells in your body, they're uniquely shaped, with a cell body, an *axon,* and branches called *dendrites.* This cell structure is needed because neurons need to communicate an immense amount of information to each other.

The transmission of this information is also unique, because it's electrical—unlike other information signals such as those sent by hormones in your bloodstream—and because these fantastically shaped neurons have one tiny little hitch. They never touch each other. Remember the space between each of them called a *synapse?* So how can neurons communicate and share their information if they don't quite touch each other?

They use a messenger service—your neurotransmitters. Neurotransmitters are chemical messengers that zap around from one neuron to another. As they're released by one neuron, this in turn stimulates other neurons, inducing a cascade of electrochemical events that produce changes in the structure of the neurons, depending on the type of neurotransmitter. This process is mind-bogglingly speedy. Synaptic connections take place in nanoseconds.

There are many different kinds of neurotransmitters in your synapses. Not only that, but your brain uses the *same* neurotransmitters in *different* areas to achieve different purposes. Take the neurotransmitter called dopamine, for example. It helps you move, and it helps you feel; in motor-function areas of the brain it's stimulated whenever you give your body a command, and in emotion-regulating areas of the brain it's used to help you modulate your feelings.

If dopamine levels are too low in the part of the brain called the basal ganglia, responsible for coordinated as well as automatic motion, your movements become jerky or uncontrollable, which is a symptom of Parkinson's disease. And if dopamine levels are too low or imbalanced in the emotional sectors, you can become depressed. (There's much more information about how neurotransmitters and exercise regulate your feelings on page 36 in chapter 2.)

The trick to achieving maximum brainpower is to get all the disparate parts of the brain to work together in seamless synchronicity. When information easily flows all over your brain, the result is better movements, better solutions to the questions you ask yourself, and better thought processes. When the information doesn't flow so easily, however, you have a brain that is out of sync. That, unfortunately, is a telltale sign of diseases or of aging, as you'll see in chapter 3.

The information flow in your brain happens in three distinct directions: back to front , left to right, and through the power of your sensory system sending information from your muscles to your brain.

First You Go Back: The Cerebellum

The cerebellum may fit into only a small area at the back of your head, but it packs a huge wallop, since 50 percent of your neurons are superconcentrated there, in only 10 percent of your brain mass. No wonder *cerebellum* literally translates to "little brain." It's like a megacomputer coordinating most of your brain's functions, especially those related to movement.

The cerebellum is responsible not just for planning and intent, but for making sure we are able to *do* what we'd planned and intended to do! As soon as it receives information from your cortex, the brain area responsible for voluntary movement, as well as from your sensory system (more on that on page 24), the cerebellum kicks into gear.

The cerebellum has three sections, each contributing something different to its overall function: one section is for posture and balance, another for coordinating movements of our arms and legs, and a third for helping us to plan our movements—what I refer to as muscle timing. It's not just a passive receiver; it needs to figure out what it is to do that will best control these balance and coordination movements. If you suffer from any kind of trauma or damage to the cerebellum, it's very likely that you'll lose at least some capacity to make coordinated movements.

The cerebellum is so special that it has its own set of distinctive and extremely complex neurons, called *Purkinje neurons*, that can process an enormous amount of information. Dr. Martin uses a lovely analogy to describe this: Compare the Purkinje neurons to an enormous tree laden with lots of branches and leaves, in far more copious amounts than other neurons. The tree trunk is like a Purkinje neuron; the branches and leaves are the receivers of all the information sent to it from other parts of the brain and nervous system.

To give you an idea of the power of the cerebellum, consider your eyes. They send information to the frontal lobes on an astonishing circuit of about one million optic nerves. Well, the cerebellum has *forty times* as many nerve fibers sending information from the back of the brain to the front!

Or consider what it takes when someone is handing you a glass of water. You instinctively know how to grab it as well as how *long* it will take you to reach out and grab it. An immature or dysfunctional cerebellum will have trouble judging this distance and timing the movements needed. This is something you see in toddlers and even in teenagers, since the cerebellum structure isn't finished developing until we're fifteen to twenty years old.

As soon as the cerebellum receives information sent from all over the brain, it processes this information and sends it right back out. When you're exercising, for example, the cerebellum fine-tunes the neural signals that determine the timing and strength of muscle contractions so your movements can be much more effective. It does this by sending specifically timed neural signals to other brain regions and making sure that the signals are the right strength.

But it does a whole lot more, too. Dr. Martin explains that as the cerebellum receives its sensory information, it doesn't function just as a passive receiver to regulate your balance and coordination. It needs to figure out how *precisely* to control these movements.

In 1995, when more than eighty studies were presented at the annual conference of the Society of Neuroscience, it was shown that the cerebellum has more functions than previously thought—nonmotor functions like speech, problem solving, concentration, attention, focusing, memory, and emotions. This is an extremely important point, because the cerebellum also fine-tunes the neural signals for speech and cognition.

So while you're exercising, you're stimulating the area of the brain that controls not only your balance and coordination, but vital cognitive functions, too. Not only does the cerebellum take in all the sensory input from our muscles and then organize it seamlessly; it also fast-tracks this information off in all directions to all other parts of the brain, particularly parts of the frontal lobes.

Then You Go Forward: The Frontal Lobes

The frontal lobes are found in the mid-front section of your brain. That's where your power decision making, problem solving, and language usage takes place. It's also the source of your powers of concentration, attention, and focus.

Whenever you start *thinking* about what you're doing when you exercise, you give your frontal lobes a good workout, too. If you just move your arm, for example, a specific area of the brain becomes activated. If you simultaneously move an arm and a leg, more areas of the brain become activated. Even better, when you instruct your brain to do a specific movement, far more areas of the brain become activated. So if I told you to raise your right leg and then do a biceps curl with your left arm, you'd have to think about it, then plan what to do—that's what I call *intent*—and only then could you follow my instructions.

That's precisely what the frontal lobes are meant to do. As soon as you hear my simple command, intent kicks in, and your frontal lobes instantly calculate with other sections of the brain the best way for you to do that leg raise and biceps curl.

This is where the power of concentration comes into play: through intent, planning, and perfect execution. This is what great athletes like Tiger Woods and Kobe Bryant do every time they think about how to move before executing the movement (although, of course, their intent/movement is superfast, thanks to their years of practice coupled with their innate skills).

For optimal brainpower, you want all the different areas of the brain triggered into activity. That way, they'll send the information that they're responsible for as quickly as possible to the frontal lobes. Then the frontal lobes take over and make the superpowerful decisions you need.

Whenever we move our arm, a few specific areas of the brain become active. When we simultaneously move an arm and a leg, more areas are activated. And when we perform an intentional action, even more areas of the brain become active. In other words, intent and planning need to interact with each other. When you intend to move with precision, your frontal lobes process the information, and the planning director that is your cerebellum does the planning.

So, for example, if you want to move both arms and your left leg at the same time, your frontal lobes recognize the intent as soon as you hear or read the command "Raise both arms and your left leg." Literally at the same time, your cerebellum will start planning as quickly as possible to convey all the information to and from your muscles via sensory feedback. Then, if the movement isn't quite right, your cerebellum will adjust, modify, and improve its execution.

Voilà! This is how a cognitive and a physical workout interact with each other, forcing the brain to think. The more you do it, the more automatic the movement becomes, which means you're ready for a more complex set of exercises that will be just as stimulating as the old ones were the first time you did them.

The Right Way to Multi-task—and No, This Doesn't Mean Talking on Your Cell Phone When You Exercise

The Super Body, Super Brain exercises are not difficult to do, but as you know by now, your brain *perceives* them as difficult, because moving so many different muscles in precisely coordinated patterns requires a lot of brain skill. What's more, the exercises demand utter (and deeply satisfying) concentration in order to be done properly. And this isn't just any kind of concentration, but a very specific kind of cognitive processing and integration of information, a process that happens without awareness and that instantaneously sends information in new ways, to different parts of your brain. Being able to quickly take in and respond to this information is what pushes your brain into hyperdrive and gives it a challenging and satisfying workout.

There's a reason for that, and it's called *focused multitasking*. It's what I asked my bored client whom I mentioned in the introduction to do. He was absolutely adept at lifting weights one at a time, but as soon as I forced him to concentrate and to combine the same old easy tasks into new patterns, his brain went from "I can do this in my sleep" to "Are you kidding me!"

According to Dr. Felice Ghilardi, a researcher and neurologist at New York University, the multitasking process in the brain consists of many different areas processing all the information and then programming appropriate outputs. Your brain does this whether it's working on a cognitive response (like solving a problem) or incorporating elements of balance and coordination with strength training to enable you to do the multitasking Super Body, Super Brain exercises.

This kind of focused multitasking is not the same as the kind you'd do if you were punching numbers into your cell phone when you're walking down the street, or reading a book while watching TV. (You're actually already unconsciously multitasking whenever you walk: your left arm swings when your right leg moves, and vice versa, right?) Such multitasking is actually counterproductive, as it decreases performance. This is because too much stimulation (book plus TV) interferes with different process centers in the brain, lessening your ability to fine-tune your concentration.

Good multitasking, however, takes skill. A fabulously focused multitasking waiter will have ten tables to manage yet instinctively know how to take care of each of them, being able to gauge when the food is ready, who needs a menu, or who needs the check. (This is both cognitive and physical multitasking.) A fabulously focused multitasking student will be able to listen to the teacher while taking notes and absorbing the information at the same time, skills that translate to doing the same thing in an office: when your boss is discussing vital information at a meeting, you're writing it down and figuring out how best to use it at the same time. And a focused multitasking exerciser will be too engaged to think about anything other than the exercise at hand. Ideally, you want the focused multitasking element to be present every single time you exercise. That way, you can be assured of maximum brainpower.

Which is why Super Body, Super Brain exercises all contain brain-zinging balance and concentration moves combined with strength training. Plus, you'll always be tweaking the movements by adding small modifications, which will activate more areas of the brain and prevent it from getting too complacent or lazy. Your brain will continuously believe that it is learning new moves, creating a spillover of activity from the motor, or muscle-controlling, centers in your brain to more diverse cognitive centers.

Stuck in the Middle with You: The Basal Ganglia, the Hippocampus, and the Striatal System

As information is flowing from the cerebellum in the back of the brain to the frontal lobes, other brain areas are stimulated as well.

THE BASAL GANGLIA

The basal ganglia, found in your brain's midsection, consist of the corpus stratium, the subthalamic nucleus, and the substantia nigra. Their function is to regulate movement coordination and voluntary and involuntary movement—our autopilot movement functions—and to actively connect to other parts of your brain, particularly the frontal lobes. (The basal ganglia are also involved in many nonmotor functions, such as attention, memory, and energy regulation.) That makes them an essential component of dealing with and improving your basic coordination.

Take walking. When a baby learns to walk, she lurches from side to side like a tipsy sailor and seems to fall down as much as she stays upright. But remarkably quickly, the walking process goes from ungainly to smooth. A baby who could barely crawl will be running all over the playground two or three months later.

So you can think of the basal ganglia as the part of the brain that helps you function on automatic pilot. You no longer need to think about how to walk—unless you've just strapped on snowshoes!

Whenever you do a new exercise routine, your basal ganglia also help you learn the movements, just as you once learned how to walk. At first, your movements are likely to be clumsy and jerky, but the more you do them, the smoother they'll become. Pretty soon, they'll be so easy to do and so fully automatic that it will be hard for you to even remember that you might once have had trouble with them.

I've structured the Super Body, Super Brain exercises to be endlessly changeable. This deliberately stimulates your basal ganglia so they can share all your newly learned patterns with the rest of your brain, strengthening its overall function and making it stronger and smarter.

THE HIPPOCAMPUS

The hippocampus is found inside the medial temporal lobe of the brain, and it is essential for learning, memory formation, and what's called *allocentric spatial processing,* or spatial navigation. This is the process that allows you to navigate in the real world so you know where you are in space and can then picture where else you may need to go.

You want your hippocampus to be as well developed as possible; the implication is that the stronger your hippocampus, the better you will be at processing memories and at being able to draw associations from unrelated items in your memories.

For instance, whenever you meet someone new, your hippocampus will help you remember that person's name by encoding it in the context of a larger episode, which would be why you met that person, and when, and where. This will help you pull up the memory should you need it in the future. These more complex, episodic memories are likely encoded by a larger network of neurons in the brain.

Eric Kandel is a neuroscientist, psychiatrist, and professor of biochemistry and biophysics at the Columbia University College of Physicians and Surgeons, and one of the most towering figures in neuroscience thanks to his studies on learning and memory. (His research on the physiological basis of memory storage in neurons won him the Nobel Prize in 2000.) According to Dr. Kandel, we have two types of memory: explicit memory, found in the hippocampus and medial temporal lobe and dealing with facts or events through conscious recall; and implicit memory, found in the amygdala, cerebellum, and reflex pathways and dealing with motor tasks or perceptual skills through unconscious recall.

According to his theories, once you master explicit memory, constant referral back to this memory allows it to move into implicit memory, because implicit memory is more efficient, going from deliberate, conscious thoughts to subconscious thoughts. In other words, the Super Body, Super Brain exercises may seem complicated at first, but once you do them consistently, you master them.

I love seeing this with my clients who've never exercised before. Suddenly, an exercise that they may have struggled with for a week is not only flawlessly executed, but is in fact too easy! That is always such an empowering moment for both of us (and it also means the client is now ready for a more complex set of exercises.)

Even more exciting, a study in the journal *Hippocampus,* as reported in *Science Daily* on March 3, 2009, claimed that "elderly adults who are more physically fit tend to have bigger hippocampi and better spatial memory than those who are less fit." This was the first new study to show that exercise can affect hippocampus size and memory in people.

THE STRIATAL SYSTEM

How do dancers learn new patterns so easily? After years of training and endless classes in which they've repeated the same movements countless times, they have a well-developed subcortical motor system called the *striatal system*. This is nonverbal, motor learning—think of it as muscle memory—which allows them to recollect a dance in the same way you can consciously recollect a conversation.

Neuroscientists believe that, possibly given a boost by the cerebellum, the striatal system develops circuits for every little move, and the interconnectedness of these circuits makes it progressively easier to learn new exercise movements and respond to commands—whether read or heard—to execute them.

Move It On Over: BrainPower from Left to Right

Your brain has two hemispheres, the left and the right, each its own universe of power. But the two hemispheres are like symbiotic twins: they can't function on their own, so they're constantly sending information from one to the other and back again so you can be a thinking, feeling person on the go.

The Left Hemisphere, the Right Hemisphere, and the Corpus Callosum

As the information flows from one hemisphere to the other and back again, it moves through a structure called the corpus callosum. The corpus callosum is like the Brooklyn Bridge connecting Manhattan with Brooklyn—and all the cars driving over it are the equivalent of your neurons.

Both brain hemispheres deal with movement. The left hemisphere of your brain controls the right side of your body, and the right hemisphere controls the left side of your body. Each hemisphere is associated with different kinds of skills: the right side of the brain is considered to be more creative, artistic, and emotional, and the left side to be more logical, analytical, and fact oriented.

There are lots of functions other than movement that require coordination of the left and right hemispheres: vision (especially three-dimensional vision and tracking objects in space); hearing; the integration of visual and verbal thinking; reading; and writing.

Traditionally, it's been assumed that someone is either right-brain or left-brain dominant, but the most current research shows that we're more likely to be a little of both and that it is very important for both hemispheres to work together and coordinate information efficiently. A perfect example would be when we're reading and understanding what we're reading at the same time.

So how can you maximize this constant side-to-side chatter when it comes to movement? Simple: train both hemispheres to strengthen their communicative powers by doing oppositional movements at the same time. That's why the Super Body, Super Brain exercises you'll do while standing always begin with this basic command: raise your left arm and right leg.

Move It On, This Time with Feeling: Brainpower, Proprioception, and Your Sensory System

Have you ever thought about *what* makes your muscles move, and *how*? I have to confess that I hadn't, even with all my sports training—until I needed to figure out why my exercises were having such a profound effect on my clients. I had to understand why our muscles move the way they do and how they are connected to our brains so I could take this information, apply it in even more depth, and maximize every movement.

I already knew that every movement we make has a purpose. It can be as simple as reaching for that first delicious cup of coffee in the morning, typing a boring report for your boss, kissing your kids' dumpling cheeks good night, or doing an exercise routine with multitasking limb movements.

And then I learned that what makes any of these movements possible is our sensory system—the component of our nervous system that deals with our senses, how we use them, where the information is processed, and how this information is sent to our brains.

The Endless Feedback Circuit and How It Makes You Move

Your nervous system has two parts: the central nervous system, or CNS, comprising your brain and spinal cord; and the peripheral nervous system, or PNS, which connects the CNS to your muscles and organs. The PNS is made up of your skeletal (somatic) system, which controls voluntary muscle movements and reflexes, and your autonomic nervous system, which regulates your breathing and heart functions. (Super Body, Super Brain targets all these systems, by the way, especially the autonomic nervous system. Proper breathing brings more oxygen to your brain, which in turn improves both brain and muscles.)

Your motor system refers to the part of the CNS responsible for movement. In fact, your body is one amazing motor system that's constantly sending information from the brain to the muscles and back again in an endless cycle of stimulation.

The CNS communicates with the PNS in two ways. First are the messages carrying information from the top down, from your brain to your muscles. These are carried along efferent, or descending, nerves.

Second are the messages carrying ascending information, from the bottom up. These come from the receptors of our sensory system in the motor neurons of our muscles, tendons, joints, and skin.

In other words, one signal comes from your brain, and the other literally comes from your body's feedback. These systems can then process the information in real time, as it's happening, since the information is needed in order for you to control how you move. And so the systems send the information back down to your muscles along your body's receptive channels, like cars driving north and south on your body's never-ending information highway. Once the signals arrive back at the motor neurons, neurotransmitters are released to activate the motor neurons. These in turn tell your muscles how to move.

This information is ceaselessly flowing in a controlled manner from down to up and back again. I like to think of it as if you were gazing down from high above Times Square. The cars are flowing into it from all directions, and the movement looks utterly chaotic at first. But then you realize that the traffic has a pattern: the stoplights are regulating the flow of the cars, and

the mojo behind motor skills

Dr. John Martin tells us, "Motor skills aren't just about being able to kick a soccer ball or hit a hockey puck. They're a crucial feature of our everyday lives and define us as humans every bit as much as our intellect or our art. Movement gives us mobility; we can choose to go where and do what we want. If our movements become hampered because of illness like a stroke or a disease like Parkinson's—we lose something important to us.

Actually, I believe that our motor skills, not our brute strength, are what got us where we are today! Just as a sharp intellect can give someone a huge advantage in business; so, too, can well-honed motor skills bring you to the top of your game. In many professions, like athletics, ballet, and surgery, the need for motor skills is obvious. So although you might not think about your motor skills, you'll certainly stop taking them for granted if you break your leg and have to hobble around on crutches, or if you're trying to fix a tiny loose screw in your only pair of eyeglasses or drive a carload of kids home in a pelting thunderstorm."

Can learning new motor-coordination patterns—what you do with Super Body, Super Brain's multitasking movements—create new synapses and strengthen existing neural connections? Neuroscientists believe it can.

You already know how the Purkinje neurons in the cerebellum process information whenever you engage in a new coordination pattern, and how they then shoot this information off to other areas of the brain. But many other parts of your motor system, particularly in your cerebral cortex, as well as the areas of the nervous system they connect to, such as the spinal cord, respond when challenged, too.

In other words, learning new coordination patterns continuously challenges all your cognitive systems. Not only are the circuits in your brain and sensory system maintained, but new connections are continually built.

The Super Body, Super Brain exercises are all designed to incorporate new coordination patterns, endlessly mixing up balance, coordination, and specifically timed muscle movements. These are deceptively complex movements. Which means that many different areas of the brain are forced to respond as they organize and process the signals they're receiving and as more brain activity is triggered. That is precisely how exercise can stimulate your brain.

what looks like a mess is actually following a logical and deliberate structure.

Proprioception Is the Body's GPS: How We Process Information from the External World

None of my clients had ever heard of the word *proprioception,* and I had a lot of fun explaining it to them. "Stand tall, raise one leg off the floor and keep it raised, and then close your eyes and clap your hands fifteen times over your head. Make sure you allow at least a second between claps," I'd say, and when they asked why, I'd simply tell them to try it.

And then they were blown away. None of them could do it with their eyes closed, even though it was a breeze with their eyes open. What had made a simple exercise so hard?

The reason is that our brains are used to relying on our eyesight; when deprived of vision, our brains are forced to compensate by using other information channels. Enter proprioception.

Proprioception is distinct from cognitive thinking or feeling. It's not something we normally think about, like listening to music, because it's so basic, even as subconscious as breathing. Derived from the Latin words (*re*)*ceptus* (the act of receiving) and *propius* (one's own), proprioception is often referred to as our "sixth sense," because it will continue to function if our other physical senses cannot.

Proprioception gives your brain information about where you are in space. Your sensory system and your proprioceptive receptors in your eyes, ears, skin, and joints constantly feed information to your nervous system, and most particularly to your brain. This tells you how to integrate information from the external world into your internal world and tells you where you are, literally, in space.

In other words, proprioception provides critical information about the position of our bodies—not just our posture but the position of our limbs. It's like having a GPS in our fingers, toes, joints, skin, eyes, and ears.

Having a good sense of where your limbs are allows you to properly control your movements. If someone is handing you a glass of water, your brain must first process the location of both the glass and the hand. Thanks to proprioception, you don't need to think about or look to see where your hand is, since proprioception is so automatic. As soon as you see the glass, you "know" exactly how far to extend your hand to take it.

Proprioception kicks in anytime you take a walk, whether on a smooth sidewalk or on a rocky beach or patch of ice (where you have to be careful of where you place your feet so you don't fall). It also snaps into alert when you raise your heels up off the ground; your body instinctively will know how high to go so you won't topple over. This is why I often have you do this kind of heel raise when you're in the middle of a Super Body, Super Brain routine.

You can test the power of proprioception yourself by going outside of your home and then closing your eyes and taking a few steps. Do you feel odd? Do you know where you are? Where can you safely move? Are you about to trip on the curb? Are you going to walk into the mailbox or another pedestrian? How far did you get, and how did you feel moving without any visual clues and cues from the outside world?

Only the blind, who've learned to compensate for the lack of proprioceptive signals to their eyes (and who still have highly developed proprioception thanks to their other senses), can navigate in a dark world. Without proprioception, you have no idea how to move or where to go.

Proprioceptive power tends to be overlooked, mainly because most people don't understand what it is. But the information flowing *up* from the receptors is as important as the information flowing back *down* from the brain. That's because proprioception is crucial not only for balance, movement, and spatial orientation, but because it's absolutely essential to use movement to integrate your proprioception with your motor system, to keep them functioning in sync since they feed off each other. Which is why I designed all the Super Body, Super Brain exercises to incorporate elements to keep your sensory system activated, using specific movements to strengthen your joints, balance, and coordination while stimulating your neural connections. And since the sensory system naturally starts to

Jill's story

"What I like best is that with Super Body, Super Brain, Michael's constantly changing it. He's always switching the exercises. We never do just one movement. It's always at least two parts, and it's always challenging. When he tells me to close my eyes and concentrate on good form and do the same amount of reps, it's another element of challenge. In my mind's eye, I'm trying to visualize what he's told me to do without asking questions, and what had been an easy exercise becomes much harder. It's a whole different skill set to do properly. After four years training with Michael, it still gives my brain a jolt.

"My body's response has also been very consistent. I'm very toned in isolated areas that needed more work. He changed the shape of my thighs. And my core is so strong. If you start doing these exercises before you have the breakdown that inevitably comes with age, I really do believe you can stave it off. They give you a great foundation of strength. And it only took about two weeks after I started for me to see results."

slow down with age, keeping it challenged with new patterns of motor coordination and movements should help keep the information flow as smooth and ceaseless as possible. This will keep you moving the way you want to as you grow older.

Get Moving and Get Smarter

Rodents might have been a scourge throughout history, but brain researchers feel more kindly toward the laboratory mice and rats so helpful to their studies. Lab rodents who had lots of toys to play with and mazes to run around in—what's called "enriched" environments—had thicker brains compared with toy-deprived, bored rats.

According to Dr. Suzuki, it wasn't the toys that made these rats' brains get so much thicker, with stronger motor-learning centers. It was the *aerobic exercise* they had as they ran around, playing with their toys as well as with each other. Regular and precise kinds of movement made their neurons bigger and with more copious connections. These playful rodents had literally changed their brain structure through exercise!

This was proven by researchers at National Cheng Kung University in Taiwan, who published the results of their study in May 2009, and the results were impressive. They'd expanded an earlier study done in the late 1990s at the Salk Institute for Biological Studies near San Diego. There, one group of mice outshone another group when trying to navigate a maze—because they'd been given running wheels in their cages, and ran around (and around!) on them all day long. The other mice didn't.

In the Taiwanese study, when the brains of these mice were examined, they had loads of new neurons. "Our results support the notion that different forms of exercise induce neuroplasticity changes in different brain regions," Chauying J. Jen, an author of the study, said.

Can Exercise Make Us Smarter?

Dr. Charles Hillman of the Neurocognitive Kinesiology Laboratory at the University of Illinois is one of the world's foremost experts on exercise and its effect on brainpower, and his landmark 2007 study was covered extensively in the articles "Stronger, Faster, Smarter" in *Newsweek* in March 2007 and "Be Smart, Exercise Your Heart: Exercise Effects on Brain and Cognition" in *Nature* magazine in January 2008, among others. His team clearly showed how aerobic exercise led to measurably improved brain function and cognition—not just in rats, but in people. And not just in healthy adults, but in adults with early signs of Alzheimer's disease such as loss of memory and cognitive ability.

One of their most compelling findings was that aerobic exercise increases the production of brain-derived neurotrophic factor (BDNF), a protein that promotes the growth of your neurons. Not only that, but these new and our preexisting neurons branch out, join together, and communicate with each other in new ways. And when our nerve connections get thicker, we're able to speed up reasoning processes.

According to Dr. Ghilardi, BDNF is active in the areas of the brain crucial for learning, memory, and higher thinking. Studies have shown how this protein may help us get smarter as well. This is what learning is all about!

Every change in your neurons and neurotransmitters shows that new information or skills have been processed and stowed away for future use. BDNF is what makes that process possible, and specific skilled movements and cardiovascular activity like the Super Body, Super Brain circuits will help you to get more of it.

More BDNF is important not just for learning but also for how well and how long your BDNF-stimulated neurons survive and function. Brains low on BDNF literally shut themselves off to new information.

This is amazingly exciting news, because if researchers can figure out how to increase your brain's BDNF levels—either with a drug or with specific kinds of exercise—then you should absolutely be able to actually make yourself smarter!

When I spoke to Dr. Hillman, he told me how the results of his study were, happily, not a surprise. Other brain researchers had already suggested an evolutionary link between physical activity and brain health—probably because our hunter-gatherer ancestors needed to be mobile and use both brain and body to capture food.

That made perfect sense to me, especially because Dr. Hillman found that aerobic exercise had a more potent effect on cognitive brain function than other kinds of exercise. Our ancestors had no choice but to *spend* energy, through heart-pumping movement, so they could survive. They didn't have the luxury of being able to take yoga classes or go salsa dancing. If they couldn't move, and move quickly, they would die.

Of course, that doesn't mean that other forms of exercise aren't good for you—only that a lot more research needs to be done on how all forms of exercise can stimulate BDNF.

What is indisputable, however, is that different kinds of movement trigger different kinds of brain activity. And learning motor skills that your brain perceives as complex requires you to think about those skills on many levels so you can successfully master them. If you want to juggle, for example, you have to learn not only how to throw the balls up in the air but also how to regulate the timing and the speed, and you have to learn all the intricate coordination moves it takes to keep the balls in motion. This would obviously require a different part of the brain than the areas that would support a more repetitive kind of exercise like running on a treadmill or pedaling a stationary bike in the gym. That kind of aerobic activity might get your heart pumping, but it's not novel enough to stimulate the brain activity you want.

I was determined to make Super Body, Super Brain as novel as possible. Ramp up the stimulation and concentration, and you're going to get the best of both worlds: strong muscles and strong brains.

I Can't Remember If You Said This, But Can Exercise Improve Memory?

One of the frustrating issues for neuroscientists is how to standardize their studies and testing. When studying memory, for instance, how can they quantify any improvements or failures in their test subjects, since each person's memory is unique to that person? Any ability to remember tasks, events, and people will vary tremendously from person to person.

And as you undoubtedly have experienced in your own life, memory can be easily affected by a host of factors. These can range from the normal aging process to hormonal changes (just ask a perimenopausal woman who's undergoing wildly shifting hormonal levels that can trigger a host of different symptoms on any given day about that!) to stress. After a horrible, taxing day at work, you're likely to forget something you've never forgotten before. So memory testing results can potentially fluctuate widely in the same person.

Despite this, some studies have been able to show that exercise *can* have a measurable effect on memory. Usually, the improvement is seen in the attention processes, which is important for learning.

ashley's story

"I was desperate to find anything that would help me with something distressing called an expressive language disorder that I have suffered with through the years. My disorder got worse as I got older—I'm now in my midforties—and sometimes expressing myself became very embarrassing to me under stressful situations, as I could not locate words.

"Unlike most people who would seek out an exercise program to lose weight and get in shape, I did this to help my brain function with the hope that my memory and my communication could be restored.

"After the first few workouts, I noticed a change. After one month, I felt like my brain had had an extreme makeover. My memory was sharp again, I could easily locate words, and my verbal communication skills were back on track."

Let's take this a step further. If you're constantly repeating specific exercise movements, can the new neural connections you'll form somehow be triggered to overlap into another section of the brain, one that might have even more cognitive functions that can help your memory?

One of Dr. Kandel's findings is that *repetition* is more important for improving neural networks than duration. In other words, how much you repeat the same task is, in the long run, better for your brain's learning power than how long you do it.

Musicians know this; they practice scales until their fingers are nimble—but if they practice scales too long they'll be super proficient at scales and stink at Beethoven sonatas. Ballet dancers also know this; they go to class every day not just to keep their muscles toned but to wake their brains up for the real work of the day—the further interpretation of the basic steps they've already done a gazillion times in class. The consistent repetition has literally drilled this knowledge into their brains, and it then becomes the basis of all future knowledge.

Learning drives us as human beings. Every time you do these Super Body, Super Brain exercises, and try to do them better, you'll be improving your neural connections. Without even realizing it, you'll have stimulated and integrated all the areas in your brain responsible for memory, movement, and higher thinking. It's the exact same process you went through when learning to ride a bicycle as a child. Even if you haven't ridden for twenty years, if you get on a bike again you'll still know what to do.

2

Every man can, if he so desires, become
the sculptor of his own brain.

— SANTIAGO RAMON Y CAJAL

The Emotional Brain and Exercise

When I was playing basketball in Spain, before every game I would take the lead and start clapping, shouting out, "Let's go! We can do it!" half an hour before every game. My energy level zoomed up until I felt perfectly and exhilaratingly ready to play, to give my very best on the court with my team.

Now, I understand that I was instinctively using energy and exercise to alter my brain chemistry. Without brain chemistry, we wouldn't be the thinking, feeling, falling-in-love humans that we are! That's because the chemicals in your brain, and the complex currents between synapses that they bring about, are what regulate how you feel, how deeply you sleep, how well you focus and concentrate, and how well you manage the usual (or unusual!) stress of your everyday life.

Most of all, once you understand the chemistry of your brain, you'll realize why you'll want to incorporate the Super Body, Super Brain exercises into your life on a regular basis. The perfect enhanced concentration you'll find yourself engaging in whenever you perform your circuits serves as the precise energetic wake-up call your brain needs—and the result will be improved attention, concentration, and precision throughout the day as well as a better mood and overall sense of well-being.

energy boost

Need to change your mood in a hurry and give yourself an energy boost at the same time? Here's a nifty trick to alter your brain chemistry in the most positive manner. It's far better to do this simple exercise than to reach for an energy drink overloaded with caffeine, sugar, and lots of other unpronounceable ingredients whenever you need a pick-me-up. It really is amazing how quickly your brain responds when you challenge it with the right commands. You can do this exercise whenever you feel sluggish during the day. It's a great way to rev up your children, too.

You need only three things: your hands, your voice, and your smile.

Your hands because you'll be clapping. The power of clapping is so powerful, it's akin to an energy explosion.

Your voice so you can use your own vocal cords to produce sounds that radiate excitement.

Your smile because you engage as many as thirty different facial muscles when you smile. Besides, smiling makes you feel good, and it makes everyone who sees you smile back.

Let's put it all together.

- From a semi-squat-plié position (as shown on page 92), with your arms down at your sides, clap between your legs.

- Stand up, and then raise your heels while simultaneously raising your arms to clap overhead. Don't forget to smile!

Reps: 10

- Every rep count should be coordinated with a loud vocal statement. You can count from one to ten or shout out positive ideas like "Let's do it," "We can do it," and "Come on."

- Do your clapping with as much speed as possible.

Exercise and Your Brain's Chemistry

"Exercise makes you feel better." Oh, sure, you've read that or been told that countless times over the years. But do you know *why* it makes you feel better?

It's all due to the cocktail of brain chemicals that help you to move, communicate, and feel just fine. One of the easiest ways to guarantee an improved balance of brain chemicals—your neurotransmitters —is through exercise. This doesn't mean you have to run a marathon. Any regular exercise schedule stimulates their release and aids in their communication with one another.

The fact that exercise improves mental health has been proven in countless studies over the years, including a fascinating study titled "Effect of Physical Activity on Anxiety and Depression," published by Presse Medicale in 2009. "Physical activity appears to be a nonspecific treatment with psychotherapeutic potential that should not be ignored." According to several experts, the way to reap maximum benefits is to exercise aerobically and to make a consistent commitment to stick to a program.

Exercise Raises Neurotransmitter Levels

I was very fortunate that my fascination with brain chemistry led me to Dr. Michael Liebowitz, founder of the New York Center for Depression and Anxiety and a professor of clinical psychiatry at Columbia University (and the Michael Jordan of psychopharmacologists). He explained to me that when we talk about brain chemistry, we're referring to the chemistry of the synapses, those spaces between nerve cells that different chemical messengers—the neurotransmitters—must leap across in order to transmit their information to other neurons.

There are approximately thirty neurotransmitters affecting our brain chemistry. Whenever you move or do any physical activity, there are several important ones that help you get where you're going. These are dopamine, serotonin, and norepinephrine.

DOPAMINE

Dopamine is similar to adrenaline and affects brain processes that regulate movement, posture, blood pressure, attention, focus, emotional response, and your ability to feel good or bad, indifferent or excited. Stimulant drugs like cocaine and amphetamines enhance dopamine activity.

SEROTONIN

Serotonin is linked to a host of critical functions and is particularly linked to the stimulation of your muscles, memory, mood, anxiety, appetite, digestion, regulation of body temperature, and sleep.

NOREPINEPHRINE

Norepinephrine is similar to adrenaline in that it helps regulate mood and manages attention, emotions, learning, and dreaming. Lower levels of norepinephrine are often associated with depression and fatigue.

Exercise Releases Endorphins

Endorphins are a unique kind of neurotransmitter. They're our brain's built-in chemical system that shields us from pain and stress and can also induce mild euphoria. These properties help explain why endorphin release is commonly called "runner's high." But the runner's high probably results from an enhancement of several neurotransmitters in addition to endorphins. Of course, you don't have to be running, or even exercising for a long time, to feel a rush of happiness: you can be doing any kind of exercise. The only hitch to endorphins is that although their release is a given during exercise, whether they'll give you that euphoric feeling every single time they're released can't be predicted.

I discussed their role with Dr. Liebowitz, who explained that endorphins are part of your brain's chemical system that work very quickly, because they are needed in cases of sudden injury and extreme stress. It's the same chemical system found in painkillers like codeine and morphine and in abused drugs like heroin.

Endorphins are good for your brain and body in many ways: they improve your immune system, improve blood circulation, have an antiaging effect by fighting free radicals, reduce stress as they help bring down cortisol levels (see page 40 for more about cortisol), and help improve your memory.

How the Power of Exercise Changes How You Feel

Exercise Helps Develop Brain Resilience

Most of us—and certainly nearly all of the people who've corresponded with me about my workouts—have bad memories about gym class. We were told we were uncoordinated, clumsy, unable to master simple movements, and just plain old klutzy. And after being told we were helplessly uncoordinated, it became a self-fulfilling prophecy.

One aspect common to most of my clients when I first start working with them is that they are constantly berating themselves about their body size or shape or (mis)perceived flaws. But after only a few sessions—when they start to feel much better and see results—little by little, they start feeling happier.

This isn't due just to pride in their accomplishments or weight loss. It's because their brain chemistry has been altered and improved. In addition, the factor of mental engagement—of fully using their mental capabilities when challenged by a complex mental task combined with aerobic exercise that keeps their heart rate up—triggers a release of powerful neurotransmitters.

The word Dr. Liebowitz uses for this phenomenon is *resilience*. Exercise can literally make your brain chemistry more resilient. The better you feel about yourself, the more resilient you're going to be in the face of adversity.

For example, if you exercise regularly and that makes you feel consistently better, your dopamine and serotonin levels are going to remain high. Those levels will remain high week after week, as long as you consistently do the work. They will increase even more when you constantly and progressively change these exercises—which is the novelty effect discussed on page 42. It's as if you're building a neurotransmitter fortress to protect yourself from incoming attacks of self-doubt or the criticism others may throw your way.

Dr. Liebowitz explored the effect of elevated neurotransmitter and endorphin levels in his fascinating book *The Chemistry of*

Love, in which he discusses the physical effects of meeting someone you care deeply about and all the classic feelings of a love attraction (butterflies in the stomach, accelerated heart rate, blushing cheeks, shining eyes, nervous gestures). Not surprisingly, the chemical reaction to falling in love can be similar to the excitement of creating a new you—one where you're not just proud of your new accomplishments but willing and able to admit how much you love this new you.

Once the small, gradual changes become more substantial and significant—which should take no more than a matter of weeks when you stick to the Super Body, Super Brain program—you will begin to feel capable of conquering and defeating those obstacles that now stand in the way of your ability to increase your self-esteem.

And this has everything to do with the neuroplasticity we discussed in chapter 1. Every time you exercise, the connections along your brain's pathways grow stronger. You may have started with the equivalent of a dirt road, which then becomes a paved road and then morphs into a four-lane highway.

In addition, you're building not only an infrastructure, but a brain language, too. You've gone from learning the exercise alphabet, to mastering words, to turning them into sentences. What might have seemed endlessly complicated and difficult at first quickly becomes the physical equivalent of reciting Shakespeare at the Globe Theatre!

Playful Exercise Makes You Feel Great

Here's another way that exercise can make you feel better: you can have fun with it. As soon as you start viewing exercise as something playful, it's no longer a chore you *need* to do—it's a joyful task you *want* to do!

I've been working for several years with the incredible Dr. Gregory Lombardo, a child and adolescent psychiatrist and expert on bipolar disorders in children, on introducing fun and play—as well as humor—into my workouts, especially those I do with children in schools around the country. In other words, we've made sure that the way these exercises are structured is playful. Not just for kids, for whom play is how they learn and is critical for their future development (an offshoot of studying how animals play, as it's how they learn the most important life lessons), but for grown-ups, who have often forgotten what a kick it can be to move! I've noticed this on countless trips to the gym, where I've seen the grim, gray faces of people trudging along on the treadmills or halfheartedly pedaling the bikes as they read a magazine. What they're doing is unwittingly sabotaging their own workouts. Not just because they're barely concentrating on their movements or their execution, but because they've forgotten all about playfulness.

Exercise Brings Structure into Your Life, Too

Something I've often discussed with my clients who have a weight problem is why they overeat when they do. They've told me that they rarely eat badly at work or with their friends or peers—that their worst eating habits invariably emerge at home, after the stress of a long day, and they just don't know what they can do to switch off the signals that lead to bingeing.

I discussed this with Dr. Lombardo, and that led us to talking about the issue of *structure*. When most people go to work, their days are structured around the tasks at hand and toward other people's expectations. But when they move from a place where their attention is focused on other people's needs to a place where there are fewer (or different) demands, those who are oriented toward service may find themselves at a loss. They get home and don't know what to do with themselves because there's no longer any structure to their time and/or tasks. Often, the first thing they do is turn on the television, a passive endeavor and a means to either escape feelings or substitute a set of programmed feelings for their authentic emotional state.

So, instead of falling into the two most addictive home activities (TV/computer and eating) as soon as you get home, try doing a structured routine like a Super Body, Super Brain circuit instead. It takes only ten minutes and can completely restructure your evening. If you can't do ten minutes, do five. Or sit quietly and meditate for five minutes. The important thing is to give yourself something good to do that provides a mental and physical disconnect from the world outside your door.

Exercise Is a Great Way to Manage Stress

Hormones are chemical messengers released by your endocrine glands to support the normal functioning of your body. These hormones regulate sexual development (estrogen, progesterone, testosterone), digestion (insulin), and stress (the corticosteroids: cortisol and epinephrine).

Stress has been hardwired into us over the millennia, likely a direct descendant of our earliest origins as hunter-gatherers, where short periods of intense stress (hunting, fear for survival) were followed by hopefully slightly longer periods of less stress/relaxation (eating after the hunt, staying in a safe environment). The need for an instantaneous jolt of energy allowing you to make a snap decision—often referred to as fight-or-flight syndrome—meant the difference between survival and a swift death.

Find yourself in a stressful situation and your brain and body instantly react, releasing a stream of cortisol and epinephrine. When they are released in response to normal stress, this gives you a coping mechanism to react to the situation at hand. Normal stress can get you energized to do an important presentation at work, to manage driving through a rainstorm in rush-hour traffic, or to make smart decisions about your life. If you've ever found yourself in a sudden surprising or frightening situation, you'll know the feeling of an instantaneous, uncontrollable jolt of energy, which can then be followed by the feeling that all the energy has literally been sucked out of your muscles, leaving you seemingly (and temporarily) paralyzed.

But there's more to stress than that. It's not just about having an instantaneous, often heated, reaction to an immediate situation. The most damaging stress is the kind that we don't even think about—the kind of stress that creates uncertainty, that is so invidious our brains can't let go of it since there's no short-term solution. This is the kind of stress that can eat at you until you literally become ill. This stress is bad for your brain, is bad for your heart, and will speed up your aging process exponentially. So, the paradox with cortisol and adrenaline is that our bodies really do need to have access to them in case we find ourselves in situations of real stress—but they're not needed for the stress we put upon ourselves. Prolonged exposure to real stress—the kind that is unrelenting, emotionally affecting, and mentally debilitating—and its attendant release of high levels of corticosteroids is what leads to stress-related problems, such as disrupted sleep, inability to focus, a short fuse, anxiety, irrational thoughts, and depression. It has been shown to directly affect many areas of the brain as well as the functioning of the neurons, particularly in the hippocampus—which is, as you know, the center of the brain responsible for memory, learning, and spatial processing.

Not only do the corticosteroids give you a jolt, elevating your heart rate, blood pressure, and respiration, but there's a physical letdown or energy crash once the situation has resolved itself. According to Dr. Liebowitz, this is actually a very dangerous time, because the most fatal arrhythmias, or irregular heartbeats, occur when you exercise vigorously, get all that adrenaline flowing, and then stop short, which is what untrained athletes might do after a race. If you don't cool down gradually, all that adrenaline—more than you need—is still circulating. So it's always better to ease out of any workout and give your heart rate a chance to get back to normal gradually.

Can you control this stress-hormone release? Sure. It's called stress management—whatever manner you choose to use so you don't get too disturbed or worried or troubled. Many people find conscious thought or breathing routines, such as yoga and meditation, to be sublimely stress reducing, which is one of the reasons that I include simple meditation techniques as part of the Super Body, Super Brain circuits, as you'll see in chapter 4 and in the routines in part 2. Finding a few minutes to meditate whenever you can is one of the best stress busters you can give yourself.

One of the primary reasons these practices that use conscious thought are so helpful is because—you guessed it—the power of positive thoughts affects your brain chemistry. You already know that your central nervous system is an electrically powerful mechanism, and every thought is a catalyst for the thought that follows it. Saying "I am strong and I am confident" will raise your endorphin, serotonin, and dopamine levels.

Saying "I am weak and stupid" will not.

The power of exercise can measurably increase the release of your endorphins while decreasing cortisol levels, which is why exercise is such a great stress reducer. If you've been under a lot of stress, you should always consult your physician prior to beginning any exercise program.

And here's something else about exercise that is often misunderstood: it can have a calming effect on your rattled nerves. Most people who've never followed any sort of regular exercise program often erroneously believe that exercise has only a stimulant effect. But that's because they consider only what happens *while* you're moving: you're sweating, you're breathing harder, you're concentrating. They don't know how great you can feel *after* you exercise. It is one of the most sublime paradoxes of movement that it is invigorating, giving you more energy, and calming at the same time.

Exercise, Anxiety, and Depression

It is a source of endless frustration for many mental health professionals that the treatment of psychiatric disorders still has so much stigma and misperception about it. Those who develop a disease like cancer or diabetes are not shunned or shamed when they seek treatment, so why should those who have a brain-centered illness be any less worthy of help? Telling someone "It's all in your head" should not be dismissal; after all, mental illness *is* all in your head—

but it's there due to inherent imbalances in brain chemistry.

Even when anxiety and depression are mild, they can have a profound effect on your quality of life. Exercise can help reduce symptoms of mild anxiety and mild depression because it raises dopamine, serotonin, and endorphin levels in your brain. Seeing and feeling the results of your accomplishment—especially seeing and feeling them so soon after starting your Super Body, Super Brain regimen—will improve your self-esteem and hopefully give you the encouragement you need to stick to the program. Keeping an exercise log will also be a helpful, tangible reminder of your progress and results. (If, however, you exercise regularly but depression or anxiety symptoms still interfere with your daily living, seek professional help. Exercise isn't meant to replace medical treatment of depression or anxiety.)

Precisely how much exercise is needed to affect these levels is not yet something that can be conclusively proven. The Mayo Clinic suggests that at least thirty minutes of exercise, at least three to five days each week, may be needed to significantly improve depression symptoms. But even smaller amounts, such as ten to fifteen minutes, which is what it takes to do one Super Body, Super Brain circuit, will help improve your mood as well as your muscles.

Dr. Lombardo, in describing how exercise can help with anxiety, says, "One of the standard expressions for anxiety is being 'uptight'—literally, because the standard reaction when someone is frightened is to tense up. What you're doing when you exercise is loosening your muscles, and that easing of muscular tension affects mood and irritability."

"It's not a magic bullet," says Kristin Vickers-Douglas, Ph.D., a Mayo Clinic psychologist, "but increasing physical activity is a positive and active strategy to help manage depression and anxiety."

Novelty and Brain Chemistry

As for novelty, Dr. Liebowitz tells us, "There are obviously different kinds of people. There are people who are highly disciplined who can do the same thing day after day and find it interesting and satisfying without any novelty to what they're doing. And there are people who lose interest and motivation really quickly. They constantly crave more novelty.

"As a psychopharmacologist, I can treat patients for depression and they can feel wonderful. And then the euphoria starts to wear off. They get used to not feeling depressed, and it's not so exciting anymore. That's true for all of us, because whatever we have, we get accustomed to, so we then want something different or something more. It's basic human behavior that's hardwired into us as a species."

The chemical systems in your brain are hardwired to thrive on change. Learn something new and exciting (or even something boring, as long as it's new!), and more dopamine will be released in your brain. That's a given.

This dopamine release creates new realities, new emotions, and new neural circuits in your brain. But here's the catch: once your wonderfully adaptable brain gets used to all this new information, it adjusts to the new dopamine level and stops getting so excited. It's as if you finally ran an eight-minute mile after training for months, and then it's no longer a challenge. You've adapted. You need a *new* challenge.

Good exercise coaches and trainers all know the need for constant challenge, which is why they often have their athletes do progressive exercises and interval training, mixing complexity, intensity, and execution in the same way that I've done with the Super Body, Super Brain exercises. Moving between different kinds of exertion and tasks not only works all your muscles but keeps your brain working, too.

This is why I've deliberately structured the exercises in part 2 on different, endlessly progressive levels. What you'll be doing is constantly changing, so you're constantly learning and concentrating. And then every four weeks you switch the exercises up, gradually building upon what you already have mastered and adding more complicated movements. This progressive structure of exercises that are deceptively simple yet seem complicated to your brain—such as moving several limbs at the same time, forcing your brain to "think"—will stimulate your brain with its perpetual and deliberate novelty so your dopamine levels remain high.

The studies done by psychiatrist, neuroscientist, and Nobel-winning (for studying how memories are stored in the brain) Eric Kandel have explored how we transform short-term memories into long-term ones—and the critical role of repetition in stimulating learning and memory. Reading about his work made me understand the process whereby my clients transformed my instructions into cognitive thoughts and then into long-term neuromuscular memory. After a certain amount of repetition, these clients no longer needed to visualize me doing the exercises; something clicked in their brain, allowing them to know what to do right away, and to do it well. This was visible proof of their brain's capacity to quickly adapt and become much more flexible.

In other words, by changing things up, you avoid getting onto one fixed pathway that then is difficult to leave. You'll have any number of paths from which to choose. And this plasticity or versatility in your brain is hardwired into how we think and process information. "There's a continual need, when you come upon a novel situation, to restructure it," Dr. Lombardo explains, "so your brain can perceive it as something that it has already experienced.

"This flexibility, or the ability to change tracks, is very important. Problems with it are something I see in children with ADD [attention deficit disorder] or bipolar disorder. A child with ADD has difficulty staying on track; a bipolar child has trouble *changing* tracks because transitions are so hard for them."

The Emotional Connection to Exercise

When my clients hire me, they invariably tell me that they want to change their bodies or lose weight. Those are laudable goals, of course—but they're leaving off something that is the most important element of any exercise regimen: the emotional component.

For me, that is key to understanding the most potent value of exercise.

If you are emotionally connected to the plan, you won't find yourself making excuses not to do it. It's far more empowering to say, "I want to be stronger and have more energy," or, "I'm doing this for my health, so I can feel better," or, "I want to be powerful." Now, with a larger goal as your mind-set, you'll always look forward to the time spent doing your routine—not only because it makes you feel so good physically and stronger mentally, but also because you're doing something good and vital for yourself. Every time you work out, you're reinforcing the fact that you deserve to look and feel good, and to have a brain firing powerfully, with improved concentration and clarity.

Still, one of the excuses trainers often hear is "I don't have time to exercise." Which is one of the reasons I designed each Super Body, Super Brain circuit to be so short. I defy anyone not to be able to find ten minutes a day to exercise!

And remember, this is not your average workout or boring run on a treadmill; it's designed to combine all those powerful brain and body systems into a harmonious yet potent punch.

It might help you to draw up a schedule and try to do your exercising at the same time each day (or at one time on Monday and another time on Wednesday, for example).

In the wonderful fable *The Little Prince*, the Fox tells the Little Prince that he must come to visit him at the same time every day. When the Little Prince asks why, the Fox tells him that it's so he can enjoy his coming before he arrives.

Setting up a particular time to do something good for yourself can help you stay motivated. Your body *and* your brain will soon become accustomed to Exercise Time—and look forward to it, as the Fox anticipates his visits from the Little Prince.

Dr. Lombardo shared this unique tip: "When I'm teaching people to breathe as a way of relaxing and not holding their breath, I tell them to practice their breathing on their way to the bathroom every time they have to go. It's not a scheduled time, but it's a time that you know is inevitable at different times during the day."

You can extend this concept to scheduling exercise during a time span when you know you'll have windows of opportunity, and casually insert your workouts into circumstances that happen all the time. This could be, for example, when the baby is napping, after the kids go to school, or when you have a midmorning break at work. And because these circuits are so short, if you miss one at the scheduled time, you can find another slot later in the day.

There is no magic formula to starting. Just bear in mind that getting off the ground will require a priming of the pump—giving yourself a consistent number of sessions to get the feel of it. It's like playing a musical instrument: Learning the new fingering patterns can be slow going, even frustrating. But then suddenly your fingers know where to go, and what had seemed at first like an incomprehensible task becomes not just easy, but deeply satisfying.

My clients have all responded to these exercises very quickly—within weeks. They all have told me how great they feel during and after each session. They don't need me to motivate them anymore: they feel so good that they can't imagine stopping. It's almost as if their brains and bodies need that constant mental challenge as well as that endorphin release, which innately helps them do it better and faster but with more grace and efficiency.

Most of all, forgive yourself if you miss some sessions. Simply go back to the beginning and start again. The worst thing you can do to your psyche is beat yourself up because you missed some sessions or ate too many cookies after a particularly trying day at work. Self-sabotage is often just as potent as self-esteem.

Another powerful option to help you commit is to make Super Body, Super Brain a family endeavor. All the exercises in chapter 12 have been designed for parents to do with their children. This gets everybody not only moving—but moving together.

Finding the Right Motivation

Unfortunately, we live in a society dominated by quick fixes and instant communication: cell phones, texting, and e-mail have revolutionized how we communicate. But there is no quick fix with exercise. And the programs touting a quick fix and superrapid results never work in the long run, because they don't teach you what to do after the initial burst. Not only that, but they often include high-impact exercises, complicated circuits, and unrealistic promises that expose untrained athletes to the real risk of injuries. For me, gradual change following a specific, easy-to-follow-and-master progression is the only way to go. That way your mind-set will gradually evolve as you master each move, giving you the impetus to continue. I was determined to design this book to be as useful to you on day 1 as on day 1001.

And here's something else to think about: it's not just about finding the time—it's about finding the right *motivation*. You have to really want, and envision, your success in order to achieve it.

This program can help you to achieve the results you want—but only if you have the right mind-set. Most important is tackling your issues from the inside out (emotionally) rather than from the outside in (concentrating only on your physical appearance). Making the decision to transform yourself because you want to feel good, have optimal health, think more clearly, manage your stress, and be strong and fit is so much more powerful than thinking that it might be nice to drop a few pounds so you can fit into that pair of jeans you've been coveting!

Furthermore, I know that you *will* lose weight if you stick to this program, so for me, that's a given. Far harder is for my clients to push past the "I just want to lose weight" state of mind to the real reasons they gained the weight in the first place. Which translates to setting up a plan and a goal, but most of all to connecting with what's really behind it: your emotional history.

Unless you acknowledge everything that made you into the person you are today, you can't move past it. But that doesn't mean you need to stay stuck in old patterns. So many of my clients age fifty and up have told me that they've never felt so powerful in their life, not even when they were in college. Enthralled, I literally watch their self-esteem and self-confidence blossom as they overcome their self-imposed obstacles and succeed at something truly remarkable. It's a hugely important, transformative personal victory.

As a result, growing older is for them no longer fraught with uncertainty. They truly believe that they're not just getting older, they're getting better—at *everything*. They've given themselves a potent sense of well-being; they're better able to manage their stress; they thrill to the achievement of the goals they've set and the transformed shape and muscles that accompany it; and they revel in their phenomenal mental and physical power.

These clients know that the circuit that goes from your brain to your muscles works

lori's story

"I was going through an especially difficult period of my life, trying to deal with the challenges of anxiety, panic attacks, and depression. I had tried several different types of workouts—plus I'd been a certified Pilates instructor so I understood the whole mind-body connection—but none of them made me feel better. And then I met Michael.

"I quickly realized that I'd been focusing on the wrong mind-set: losing weight because I wanted to be a smaller dress size instead of dealing with what really counted in my life. Michael made me understand the importance of the emotional program attached to the physical program. Once that sank in, I was able to throw all my energy toward the right set of goals and stop sabotaging myself.

"Once we started working together, I lost a tremendous amount of weight very quickly. But more important to me was the fact that I felt so much better, particularly with my work. I'm a professional chef. I could be cooking at dinner parties for sixty people and supervising all my staff, and the anxiety about how to manage and multitask could do me in.

"When I do the routines, I feel as if I'm in what I call 'the flow.' Every move flows into the next, and it's incredibly soothing. But at the same time it's empowering and energizing. For me, these exercises are as important for my mental health as a pill. Plus, the only side effect they have is to make you look better and feel better—which does wonders for your self-esteem!"

with less dexterity as you grow older—particularly if you don't exercise at all. And they're determined to stay on top of their game for as long as possible.

Once you regularly do exercises that incorporate strength training, balance, and coordination, the new coordination patterns will fine-tune your brain.

Which brings me back to brain chemistry, and all those one hundred billion neurons in

your brain—neurons that I like to think of as a basketball team. Each neuron is a player, and the neurotransmitters are the basketball they dribble across the court. But as you know, the players can't touch each other, so they make new connections by passing the ball from one player to another via the synapses in order to make the basket.

Indulge me in this metaphor. After all, who would you prefer to have in your head? A team that will fight to win the championship or a team that has no aspirations larger than a halfhearted pickup game followed by an evening celebrating at a local dive?

I know which team I'd choose—the one that learned how to incorporate cognitively and physically challenging exercises in unique combinations to improve their brains and their bodies. Best of all, it's never too late to join this team, because the stronger the connections and teamwork you form in your brain, the more powerful your brain is going to be.

3

Lack of activity destroys the good condition of every human being, while movement and methodical physical exercise save it and preserve it.

—PLATO

Exercise and Your Health

N ow I know what 'Feel the burn' means," my forty-nine-year-old client Amanda ruefully told me several years ago, "because I'm feeling it in my knees every day!"

The lovely Amanda was yet another victim of the hard-pounding aerobics craze of the 1980s, where she happily sweated off her day's stress in one step class after another. Like so many other high-impact-loving aerobicizers, she had unwittingly been setting herself up for premature (and often progressively severe) joint damage, particularly in the hips and knees, decades later.

So I became determined to create an exercise system that would first of all demand powerful concentration, so that you can think only about proper movement execution and proper posture alignment, powering up your brain with multitasking balance and coordination movements, but that would also give you brain-strengthening benefits—and heart- and lung-strengthening cardiovascular benefits, too.

Why We Need to Exercise

Why is exercise so important for a healthy brain and body? A landmark study, published in the *Journal of the American Medical Association* in February 1995, showed clear evidence linking even small to moderate amounts of physical activity—what the researchers said was the equivalent of brisk walking at three to four miles per hour for most healthy adults—to measurable health benefits. The intent of this study was to try to convince American adults to become more physically active.

This study proved that physically active adults, when compared with sedentary adults, were able to better protect themselves from the risk of several chronic diseases, including coronary heart disease (CHD), hypertension, osteoporosis, non-insulin-dependent diabetes, colon cancer, and anxiety and depression.

In addition, researchers found that "exercise training improves CHD risk factors and other health-related factors, including blood lipid profile, resting blood pressure in borderline hypertensives, body composition, glucose tolerance and insulin sensitivity, bone density, immune function, and psychological function." On the other hand, those who were sedentary had a higher death rate, with estimates that as many as 250,000 deaths per year in the United States were attributable to a lack of regular physical activity.

Exercise Is Good for Your Heart

Risk factors for heart diseases, including hardening of the arteries, include high blood pressure, cigarette smoking, high cholesterol, diabetes, being 30 percent above your ideal weight, and/or a family history of heart attacks before age fifty-five in men and before age sixty-five in women. This is not information to ignore. According to the American Heart Association, over one-third of the adult population in the United States is at risk for cardiovascular disease, with over 409,000 men and over 454,000 women dying from it every year.

One of the indicators of optimal cardiovascular health is to have few if any signs of inflammation in your blood vessels. Ideally, you want your blood vessels to dilate easily, keeping inflammation to a minimum, so that you can have optimal blood flow to your brain, muscles, and all other tissues.

The more you exercise, the more you lessen your body's inflammatory response. Plus, the better the oxygen intake in your tissues will be. This is extremely important, because when your tissues' oxygen intake increases, your lungs are able to take in more oxygen and process it and send it to your cells more efficiently.

Furthermore, the more you exercise, the more nitric oxide your body produces. As a result, your blood vessels are less "sticky," which is what attracts cholesterol deposits.

In addition, exercise strengthens not just your heart but the peripheral muscles as well, particularly as their ability to use oxygen improves. Your basic energy level increases as a result.

When my clients started doing their Super Body, Super Brain circuits, they'd be sweating right away, so I put heart-rate monitors on them to check their pulse. Their heart rates were up, but they never went higher than the target goal of a moderate, aerobic level. Simply by doing exercises combining balance and coordination, they were able to work an incredible amount of muscles at once, which required full-on cardiovascular activity.

Exercise Can Help Prevent Type 2 Diabetes

In the last few decades, the incidence of type 2 diabetes has been increasing at terrifying rates. According to the American Diabetes Association, nearly twenty-four million American adults and children have diabetes, but nearly one-quarter of them are as yet unaware of it. Even more shocking, nearly fifty-seven million people have prediabetes. What's even more terrifying is that many cases of type 2 diabetes are wholly preventable.

Diabetes is caused by irregularities with insulin, the hormone secreted by your pancreas. Its function is to regulate the metabolism of sugar and starches and convert them into usable energy by the body. But when too much sugar is consumed—in the form of the simple carbohydrates (white bread, white sugar, pasta, juice, and so on) that are the primary sources of most calories for most people—insulin can't properly regulate it, leading to spikes in blood sugar that prevent cells from working properly and serious complications including circulatory disorders and organ failure.

There are two types of diabetes: type 1, which is not preventable because it's genetically triggered; and type 2, which is caused primarily by lifestyle and genetic predisposition. Few people who eat a nutritionally sound diet, have a normal weight, and exercise regularly develop

instantly bring down your blood sugar

After every meal, go for a ten-minute walk or do the following exercise.

- Stand tall, both arms at your waist, holding either light hand weights or bottles comfortably in your hands.

- Do a biceps curl (see page 128) with your left arm while raising your right leg, and then repeat with the other arm and leg. This is one rep.

Reps: 50–100

type 2 diabetes. Those who are overweight and sedentary do.

I have been collaborating with one of the largest pension funds in America to help their members with diabetes learn how to incorporate Super Body, Super Brain into their daily routine. Diabetics are at grave risk for life-threatening complications with their circulation, leading to amputations, blindness, and death, so it is crucial for them to get up and move.

As you'll see, exercising for short periods three times a day can be as effective as one longer workout. Frequent exercise may be particularly beneficial for diabetics, as was shown in a 2007 study done in Denmark and published in the journal *Diabetologia*. In this study, researchers concluded that breaking up the exercise sessions meant that the total energy expenditure was higher after three short workouts than after one longer workout, and that the higher energy expenditure helped subjects manage blood sugar more effectively.

Exercise Can Help Prevent Metabolic Syndrome

Metabolic syndrome is the name for a group of medical disorders that put you at higher risk for developing cardiovascular disease or diabetes. According to the American Heart Association, it has become increasingly common in the United States, with an estimated forty-seven million adults suffering from it. That's because the criteria include having a large waist circumference (forty inches and up for men and thirty-five inches and up for women), high cholesterol, high blood pressure, and other factors.

Exercise Can Help Lessen Bone Loss, Manage Arthritis, and Prevent Osteoporosis

Another great thing exercise does is make your bones more dense. Weight-bearing exercise like walking, dancing, tennis, low-impact aerobics, and, of course, Super Body, Super Brain is something everyone needs to add to their regular exercise routine if only to help lessen bone loss that is inevitable with age, particularly with post-menopausal women who no longer have the bone-protecting power of estrogen in their system. (Adding estrogen postmenopause with hormone-replacement therapy is no longer recommended because it is a risk factor for developing breast cancer.)

The catch is that this exercise has to be done regularly (three or four times each week for at least thirty to forty minutes) in order to maintain these benefits for your bones. Without constant use, muscle fibers atrophy; lower muscle volume is accompanied by a decrease in bone density. Weak bones become brittle and easier to fracture and are thus a huge fear among the elderly, because a simple fall can have catastrophic results for them. Strong bones and muscles, coupled with exercises that improve balance and coordination, provide extra insurance for all bodies as they grow older.

The right kind of exercise can also help with either osteoarthritis (caused by a breakdown of the cartilage in the joints) or rheumatoid arthritis (caused by inflammation of the lining of the joints). Workouts that are nonimpact and of moderate intensity, that increase your range of motion, and that build strong muscle around the joints to give them additional support are extremely beneficial.

The good news is that you can do something about these diseases by deciding to take care of yourself. One of the reasons I designed the Super Body, Super Brain exercise circuits to be so short is that anyone and everyone can find the time to do them, as you'll see in the next section.

Save Your Joints

Anyone who spent any time exercising through the 1980s will have an indelible memory of a sleek and svelte Jane Fonda in her striped leotard, exhorting her aerobics students to "feel the burn."

Feel the burn they did—until they burned out.

As reported by David Sheff in the *New York Times* on February 8, 2007, in the article "Whatever Happened to Jane Fonda in Tights?" a spokesman for the Sporting Goods Manufacturers Association said that from a peak of seventeen to twenty million happy aerobicizers in the 1980s, the numbers fell tremendously to under five million in 2005 and are continuing to drop. The reason is simple: injuries from all that repetitive pounding, especially to the joints of the legs, took many years to show up, but when they did, the results were dire: knees needed to be replaced.

We all know that the more you move, the more calories you burn. But the more you move, the more you can stress your joints, particularly your knees and ankles, and particularly if you are overweight. For example, if you weigh 130 pounds and go out for a nice long run, take a step class, or play basketball, every time you take a step, 130 pounds is shifted onto one leg and then the other. If you weigh 230 pounds, all that weight will be shifted from one side to the other with more impacting results. If your muscles are not strong and conditioned to take the impact, your joints will be more exposed to injury.

But if exercise has such a positive impact on our brains, why shouldn't we engage in sports as much as we possibly can? Well, the most important reason is that doing any kind of regular sport requires joint impact and sustained rotations, which often leads to injuries much more quickly than if you were doing slow, controlled, varied movements. In addition, doing any sport involves skill, and not everyone has the skills necessary for the sport they might be interested in. Plus, certain sports are not aerobic, so they don't up your heart rate or burn very many calories or fat. You need only look at weekend golfers to understand that although playing golf may be enjoyable, it is not high on anyone's weight-loss list!

A far more effective way to increase your heart rate and burn calories without putting that extra weight on your joints is by doing balance and coordination exercises with combined strength training—the essence of the Super Body, Super Brain program.

Weekend warriors who exercise on an irregular basis often don't realize how much intense training, with nonimpact exercises, professional athletes do in the off-season to help prevent injuries all year round. As a result, weekend warriors often get injured after doing high-impact cardio because they haven't balanced out their routines with other exercises that strengthen tendons, ligaments, and muscles.

This doesn't mean you need to give up the cardio exercise you love and that likely helps you manage your stress. If you are close to your ideal body weight, have developed a strong core, and have added elements of balance and coordination to your routine, your body will be stronger and better able to absorb some of the impact. What I do is combine my daily Super Body, Super Brain circuits with several days of cardio, including the basketball games that I love with a passion. A similar schedule would likely work for you, too.

rebecca's story

"I'm a yoga instructor, and when I was pregnant with my second child I'd gotten gestational diabetes and gained an unbelievable one hundred pounds. At first I went to a fancy NYC gym, but all the trainer did was put me on the treadmill, even after I'd said that I'd just spent forty-five minutes walking my older son to school and was already warmed up! Plus I have knee issues, so I could not do anything remotely high impact.

"Michael's program was exactly what I was looking for. We met three times a week in my apartment, and he tailored his workout for my goals—no impact, and my need to lose the baby weight. I lost twenty pounds, then forty more, and the last ten took a while. So the biggest challenge was to devise exercises that give me the effects of high-impact exercise without actually doing anything high impact!

"The leg movements don't go past a ninety-degree angle, so my knees and other joints are always protected. And I also liked how the movements come out of your everyday repertoire of movements. There's nothing you can't easily do—but the combinations and multitasking are what's unique.

"When I used a trainer to guide me in the gym, I felt tight, stressed, and bulky. But these exercises are ideal for someone who does a lot of yoga: they made me even more pliable. It's as if my body has become more spacious and not compacted. Instead, it's toned, lean, and flexible."

SUPER BODY SUPER BRAIN

Working Out at Medium Intensity Is the Way to Go

Typically, we're told that we must exercise at least three to five times each week, for at least thirty to sixty minutes per session, in order to see any physical or health results. But one of the worst mistakes people make when they want fast changes is to increase their cardio, doing some form of high-impact, high-intensity exercise over a sustained period, such as running on a treadmill or taking an aerobics class for an hour, coupled with an intense weight-lifting regime, all while drastically cutting calories. Of course there are benefits to training at a high intensity, particularly to strengthen your heart and muscles. But for the average exerciser, not only can high intensity cause injuries—it can cause burnout. If you give up exercising in frustration because you can't sustain a tough level of workouts, then it's no good to you at all.

And on the other end of the exercising spectrum is a colleague at the investment bank where I used to work. He was fond of telling me that he just didn't have time to exercise for an hour—so why bother at all?

The latest research shows that breaking up the workout sessions may have the same cardiovascular and pulmonary result, or one that's even better.

According to a Stanford University research study, three ten-minute workout sessions (morning, lunch, and evening) produced the same benefit as one solid thirty-minute workout. The benefits of increased peak oxygen uptake—weight loss and a lowering of the heart rate—were virtually the same in both test groups. The reason three ten-minute workout sessions might improve your benefit is that in the one-time-per-day group, there was only one cooldown—the period during which the heart rate stays elevated for a half hour after exercise. Which means that if you exercise three times a day, you have three cooldowns and thus three periods of guaranteed elevated heart rate.

The key, as with so many other things in life, is moderation. Sure, it's nice to have meandering walks with a friend (easy, slow workout) or to challenge yourself and run until you're dripping with sweat on the treadmill (hard, fast workout). But the most efficient, effective way to burn the fat stored in your body is by training at a *medium* intensity level while you're multitasking and confusing your muscles, working your brain and your sensory system at the same time. During this kind of workout, you will deplete your fat stores before you've depleted your muscle tissue, which can happen for those who train at high intensity for long periods without sufficient calorie consumption.

And because exercising at medium intensity gives you proven health benefits, you can change the exercise from good to great by doing strength training with hand weights while staying in constant motion. This will not only help your heart and lungs but make you leaner and stronger. The best way to ensure a medium-level workout is through strength training and circuit training, which extensive research has shown to be extremely effective at reducing body fat while increasing lean muscle mass.

When you do the Super Body, Super Brain circuits, you will be working out at a medium intensity while engaging dozens of muscles at the same time—still reaping the rewards of maximum power in a compressed time period without overtaxing your body. It's quality time, not quantity time!

Aerobic vs. Anaerobic Exercise

There are two kinds of exercise: aerobic (bringing in oxygen) and anaerobic (giving out oxygen). Both have their benefits, which is why athletes do varied workouts incorporating different elements for maximum results. Aerobic exercise is done at a moderate rate, and with the presence of oxygen. The Super Body, Super Brain exercises can get you up to your target zone in less than a minute. Then you'll have time to catch your breath and get your strength back for the next sequence.

The easiest way to figure out for yourself whether you're training aerobically is to determine whether you'd be just about able to maintain a conversation while exercising. This is because when you're training aerobically, your body has enough time to process the oxygen from outside, inhaling

find your target heart rate

Age	Target Heart Rate Zone (55–75 percent of maximum heart rate) (in beats per minute)
20–29	100–150
30–39	95–142
40–49	90–135
50–59	85–127
60–69	80–120
70+	75–113

Karvonen Formula Steps
1. Subtract your age from 220.
2. Check your resting heart rate.
3. Subtract that from the figure in step 1.
4. Multiply that number by 65 percent for your low range and by 85 percent for your high range.
5. Add the resulting figures to your resting heart rate. That will give you the low end and the high end of your target heart rate.

My Target Heart Rate
220 − 34 = 186
46 (yes, my heart rate is that low!)
186 − 46 = 140
140 x .65 = 91 (low range)
140 x .85 = 119 (high range)
91 + 46 = 137
119 + 46 = 165

My target heart rate = 137–165.

it into your lungs and spreading it throughout your entire body. The more oxygen you bring in, the more efficiently your heart and lungs work in sync. This strengthens the sides of your heart, leading to a slower and more efficient resting heart rate. In addition, working out at this level is close to the frontier separating aerobic and anaerobic, where your heart rate is at 65 to 75 percent of its maximum level. This is the stage at which you are most likely to have that lovely endorphin release, giving you a runner's high.

Ten Minutes of Exercise Three Times a Day Can Be as Effective as Exercising for Thirty Minutes at One Time

When the Centers for Disease Control and Prevention (CDC) released its sedentary-lifestyle death rates back in 1995, those were shocking figures. What's even more shocking, though, is that obesity rates have skyrocketed since that study was released. One of the primary reasons was that, according to the CDC, over 60 percent of American adults were not regularly active, and 25 percent were not active at all. Why is that? Because most people erroneously believe that "to reap health benefits they must engage in vigorous, continuous exercise." The CDC's recommendation was that all adult Americans should work out for at least thirty minutes, doing some form of moderate-intensity physical activity, nearly every day—and preferably every day.

Even more important for the Super Body,

Super Brain program, these recommendations not only encouraged everyone to reap the benefits of moderate-intensity physical activity, but showed how intermittent activity, breaking up the recommended thirty minutes of activity into short bouts, was also extremely beneficial as long as it was done with the same intensity you'd have as when you'd take a brisk exercise walk.

"These unique elements of the recommendation are based on mounting evidence indicating that the health benefits of physical activity are linked principally to the total amount of physical activity performed," the CDC study claimed. "This evidence suggests that amount of activity is more important than the specific manner in which the activity is performed (i.e., mode, intensity, or duration of the activity bouts)."

The importance of this study cannot be underestimated, because it clearly proved that you don't need to go to a gym and do a hard hour of cardio exercise every day in order to improve your health.

Even better, you won't just help your heart—you'll be triggering the release of the good neurotransmitters, particularly dopamine, serotonin, and endorphins, so you'll feel good three times more often. This can be particularly beneficial for anyone dealing with a lot of stress.

"I think that breaking up your exercise sessions is a brilliant idea also for stress management, blood circulation, and sleep management," Dr. Nelly Szlachter, a gynecologist who treats many women who have menopause-related problems, told me.

"Moreover," the CDC study added, "for people who are unable to set aside 30 minutes for physical activity, shorter episodes are clearly better than none."

In other words, exercise that raises your heart rate and trains you aerobically is good for you.

Furthermore, most of the cardiovascular scientific data indicates that what counts is not the intensity of the workout but its regularity or consistency over time. You want to aim for at least sixty to one hundred minutes each week, which is as little as ten minutes six times a week for beginners, gradually increasing to one hundred minutes each week once you're accustomed to exercising.

Dr. Brad Radwaner, a cardiologist and founder of the New York Center for Heart Prevention and Disease, also suggests that those who are significantly overweight (with a body mass index, or BMI, over 25) or obese (BMI over 30) need more time to exercise, either per week or per session, with a minimum of twenty minutes three times a week. Those looking to lose twenty to fifty pounds should exercise at least four or five times each week.

Gradually incorporating physical activity into your daily routine can benefit anyone who's gotten approval from their doctor to do so. One study by the Cooper Institute in Dallas, undertaken from 2001 to 2006 involved 464 women who were sedentary, postmenopausal, and overweight or obese. Not surprisingly, all women who added movement to their lives saw improvement, even those who moved the least. They felt better and had more energy.

The potential that we all have is incredible. However, to reach that potential, we need to be consistent, disciplined, and hungry to achieve the myriad benefits. You hold this power. It is up to you.

4

Physical fitness is not only one of the most important keys to a healthy body, it is the basis of dynamic and creative intellectual activity.

—JOHN F. KENNEDY

Super Body, Super Brain
Putting It All Together

One day, many years ago, I was working with my client Jody in the gym, carefully watching as she did her circuit on the weight machines. Her eyes suddenly widened; then she shook her head and said, "What a waste."

"What do you mean?" I asked her.

"I mean that lady over there, on the bike," she said, tilting her head toward the rows of recumbent bicycles. There sat a woman, barely pedaling while deeply engrossed in a magazine. "Why does she even bother?"

It was an excellent question, and one I've often gone back to as I devised the exercises in this book. What I wanted to do was create an exercise routine that would always engage your attention, so that you'd never just be going through the motions as that woman on the bicycle was doing. Every time you do a circuit, you'll be sweating and your heart will be pumping, but you'll be exercising in a precisely controlled manner so that you'll experience maximum cardiovascular benefits as well as burn the most fat in the shortest possible time, without impacting your joints. And since these exercises are progressive, you'll not only maintain your strength but keep improving without ever getting bored.

Combining high repetitions with low weights gives you the best of both worlds: an aerobic workout as well as strength training during your circuits, as you'll see in part 2. Circuit training is one of the most effective ways of reducing body fat while increasing lean muscle mass, which raises your metabolism and automatically burns more calories. Plus, if you follow a strength-training program that alters your body fat, you'll get the body you've always wanted, and you will *not* put the weight back on!

There are many unique elements to the Super Body, Super Brain program, so read on for details about what makes it so special.

About Balance: The Importance of a Strong Core

Core is one of those exercise buzzwords thrown around with a lot of misperceptions. Most people erroneously think that their core consists of their abdominal muscles, and that endless crunches will get them a nice flat belly (if they're a woman) or a six-pack (if they're a man). Sadly, doing crunches and not much else for your core will get you some aching muscles in your belly and a stressed-out neck and lower back. In fact, I see crunches as strictly old-school training that will hopefully disappear along with "feel the burn," to be replaced by a more integrated approach that treats all the core muscles as a whole.

I've seen this with nearly every one of my clients, who come to me with a weak core even though many of them have been exercising for years. Because their core muscles were actually underdeveloped, they felt this weakness on the opposite side of their body: in their lower backs. They often felt a tightness there, sometimes so achy, with the ache even radiating down their legs, that they had to lie down to make the twinges go away.

Your core is actually a much larger area, running from your breastbone down to your pelvic area. And it's not just your front; instead, it should be thought of as three-dimensional, including your sides and your back as well for a total of twenty-eight different muscles.

Think of your core as your body's powerhouse. It gives you solid strength. That's why those who do exercises that give them a strong core usually find that their lower-back pain disappears along with their soft bellies.

Balance and Your Core

If you've done crunches to no avail, you already know how tricky it is to develop a truly strong and toned core. Frankly, having a six-pack is no indication of core strength, either—only of well-developed muscles in the front of your body.

One easy way to see if your core is strong is to bend one knee and lift that leg up, then touch your stomach with one hand. What do you feel? Is it hard? In that position, your core muscles are engaged because they need to stabilize your balance.

Another way is to stand tall, arms spread wide, and then bend your left knee and touch your left ankle with your right hand. Can you do that without losing your balance?

Instead of crunches, try balance training.

Anytime you incorporate balance exercises into your workout, you're automatically engaging all your core muscles at the same time, as you need them to stabilize your body. All the Super Body, Super Brain exercises are a variation of a powerful strength-training movement combined with balance movements, whether you're at Level 1 or Level 4 or beyond. Advancing to a higher level is a sign of core strength more than anything else is!

And don't forget that one of the most important aspects of balance is the amount of brain activity that it stimulates. Balance is an instant trigger of the proprioceptive receptors of your sensory system, as you learned in chapter 1. Every time you train your core properly, the information flow to and from your brain kicks into overdrive.

Coordination and Timing

I use the word *coordination* a lot because it's another one of those exercise buzzwords that is sorely misunderstood. Coordination is not something that only trained athletes like dancers, gymnasts, and figure skaters possess. As you know already, if you can walk, you're coordinated! But most people

Indran's story

I met Indran, a forty-two-year-old management consultant, when I worked as a trainer at New York Sports Club. He had a slipped disc back injury, which happens when the discs that act as cushions between the vertebrae become dislodged, causing friction in the bones. The catalyst had been the countless hours he spent sitting hunched and crouched in front of his laptop, coupled with playing field hockey almost every Sunday since he was a little boy. Pains were shooting down to his ankle on his left side, and he could no longer play hockey—a devastating blow. Physical therapy offered no relief, and his physicians suggested he give up sports altogether. But he wouldn't bow out without a fight.

I started training with him three times a week, helping him strengthen the core muscles of his abdomen and surrounding his spine. Within six months, his back pain had subsided and Indran was back on the hockey field. A year later, he revisited one of the doctors he'd seen before starting my program for an MRI. There was his formerly slipped disc, comfortably tucked back into alignment. His doctor was flabbergasted. That's the power of a strong core!

andrea's story

"I met Michael when my husband and I hired him for only one hour, to teach us how to use the equipment that had just been installed in the gym in our apartment building in New York, but after one session we were hooked!

"At the time I was in my midforties and my shape had been shifting as I put on weight in my middle, and I was afraid my brain was going to turn to mush, as a lot of my girlfriends had warned me about. Instead, I was more energetic, stronger, and balanced, walking tall down the street with confidence because I was so strong in my core. Years of chronic shoulder pain also disappeared, which I'm convinced is due to my toned and firm shoulder and upper-back muscles that gave me extra strength where I'd really needed it.

"I really noticed this when I went hiking again. It was an activity I'd done a lot when I was in my twenties, but I gave it up as I got older and felt more unsteady on my feet. I lost my nerve, and I was too timid and uncertain on rough terrain to enjoy those hikes anymore. But, suddenly, there I was on the trail, not afraid anymore thanks to my new powers of balance and coordination."

I've trained are convinced they're hopelessly uncoordinated, when of course they aren't. They just think they're incapable of putting deceptively simple movements together in an effective sequence because they've never been taught to do so.

Simply put, coordination is anything that you do requiring different muscle groups and parts of your body to work at the same time or with specific timing per your mental instructions. It can be as simple as raising your arms when you move your legs to stand up to give a concert pianist a standing ovation. It can be walking. It can be playing a sport that involves hand-eye control, like tennis, golf, or playing catch with your kids.

Coordination is possible because it is an essential brain function. In addition, the left side of the brain controls the right side of the body, and vice versa. Whenever you lift your left arm and your right leg, you're doing a coordinated movement that involves the transmission of information between both right and left brain hemispheres. In other words, you're using your entire brain.

Proper breathing improves the quality of the movement and also increases the oxygenation that sends blood to your muscles. You'll learn how to breathe more effectively later in this chapter.

Timing is also an essential element of coordination. Timing involves precision of thought as different parts of your body move in simultaneous yet different sequences toward a goal. (This is why tennis looks so easy until you try it for the first time and can't even hit the ball.) When we incorporate timing, we force our brains to process the intention, plan the movement, and then execute it with precision—all in a matter of milliseconds.

You don't need to be an athlete to have superbly coordinated timing. Every time you get in and out of a car—or open a tube of toothpaste, squeeze some out, then brush your teeth—you're using motor skills, timing, and coordination to get the task done seamlessly.

Flexibility and Strength

When I tell my clients that flexibility and strength go hand in hand, they usually look at me as if I've just sprouted another head! To them, flexibility means being able to stretch themselves into a human pretzel in yoga class, or some magical quality that gymnasts have as they do triple flips in the Olympics. It's something they're convinced they'll never have (like coordination).

Flexibility is one of the most powerful elements of fitness in our lives—and one of the most overlooked. Put simply: it means that you're able to have a very wide range of motion so you can activate a specific muscle group on command and extend it

where you want it to go without feeling tension or tightness. A muscle is in perfect shape if it's firm and taut, both extremely flexible and extremely strong.

Muscles are meant to be used; as a species, humans are wired to be in constant motion. (Think about this the next time you're unconsciously tapping your fingers or swinging your legs during a boring meeting.) Our muscles are bundles of wide muscle fibers that need to be strong and pliable in order to work effectively. Activate them and they expand like an inflated balloon, which is a good thing. If you've ever seen a drawing of your muscles in an anatomy book, they look strong and lean.

But for most people, that depiction is inaccurate. Without regular use, muscle fibers change shape, start to atrophy, and shrink into a knotted, dense ball, since they're no longer getting the extension and contraction that should be keeping them flexible.

Without flexible muscles, your joints are far less protected and gradually become more prone to injury. When a professional football player gets tackled, the more flexible and strong the player's joints, the less likely they are to break with each impact. It's like a tree bending in the wind. Even the strongest tree will break if the force upon it is too strong, but a tree that bends and moves is able to absorb and dissipate the shock. Eventually, though, the less you use your muscles, the more they atrophy until you get to the point where it's actually hard to move, and the less they can surround and protect your joints and bones, making a fall more likely to result in a fracture. Fortunately, anyone can regain some degree of flexibility in their muscles with regular use, no matter what their age. I always tell my clients that the less flexible their muscles, the more that will speed up the "shrugging process"—what happens to people, particularly in their fifties, when they store mid-body fat, jiggling whenever they shrug. If, however, you activate the oblique muscles, they expand, and eventually the shrug will disappear. Not only that, but strong and flexible obliques make you taller, because you will be standing much more upright with their firm support. One of my clients, who was the same height as I am when we started working together, is now taller than I am—which he is fond of mentioning whenever we meet!

Your goal with Super Body, Super Brain isn't to be a gymnast, but to have your body function in the way it's supposed to and always allow you to perform the tasks you ask of it. Every Super Body, Super Brain movement has been designed to improve your flexibility; every movement consists of shortening (muscle tension) and lengthening (flexibility). With, for example, a simple semi-squat plié with an upper-back extension, first you contract (shorten) your legs and bend (shorten) your arms, and then you extend (lengthen) arms and legs to increase your flexibility, making your muscles longer and leaner through repetitions in a specific range of motion. That's true flexibility.

Only after regaining flexibility will you be able to see rapid improvement. When my clients start to work with me, about 70 percent of the work I do with them is

flexibility stretches

- Stand tall, legs wider than shoulder width apart, arms out to the sides at shoulder height, and then reach down to your knees. Stand up and stretch your arms backward while looking up at the ceiling and saying a huge "Ahh."

- Stand tall, legs wider than shoulder width apart, and then place both hands behind your neck and lean completely to one side while breathing normally. Hold for ten seconds, and then repeat on the other side.

to improve flexibility, and 30 percent is to develop strength. After about two weeks, the percentage shifts to about 50–50, eventually ending up at 70 percent strength and 30 percent flexibility, which I believe is the perfect ratio. That's because your muscles can't be strong until they've been trained to be flexible. My Super Body, Super Brain program takes you on this same path to strength and flexibility.

Progressive Training: Train Like the Pros

When I was a child growing up in Spain, basketball was my passion. One concept that has stayed with me since my basketball days is the idea of mixing up training routines: my team was always coached to work out differently at the start of the season than during the ready-to-win-the-championship push at the season's climax. Our coaches knew that we had to mix it up—to do specific, progressive exercises to constantly challenge our bodies, to keep our muscles strong and our brains focused on the game.

In the preseason we would start slow, with long endurance sessions to condition our hearts and muscles. Gradually, we moved on to more interval and power training as the season progressed. At the time, one of my coaches made a deep impression on me. "Don't think all this training is just to make you strong," he said, "because it's not. It's to keep you from getting injured.

If you're going to play a high-impact sport, you need to have a progressive conditioning program so you'll gradually get stronger and stay strong so you won't get injured."

I became determined to apply his same philosophy to the Super Body, Super Brain program. A structured progression is essential. After all, progression is how we learn and master any new skill so our neuromuscular system will adapt to it. Teachers have a curriculum for the entire year, because they know that their students won't be able to read unless they first learn the alphabet, then little words, then sentences, then paragraphs. Everything you learn builds upon your prior knowledge. I don't really understand those programs that have no progression and just promise long-lasting results with a set of exercises.

Another important reason to mix things up is that gradual change is sustainable—and as you know, Super Body, Super Brain is a program for life. Sure, gyms are supercrowded in January with exercisers determined to live up to their New Year's resolutions. But how many of these gymgoers are there four months later?

With these exercises, the movements take place in a deliberately structured sequence incorporating balance, coordination, joint and muscular strength, and cardiovascular activity into one seamless whole. You'll first master each level and then gradually move on to exercises that build upon what you've already grown accustomed to doing. Progressive training gives you powerful cardiovascular conditioning; it's athletic

surprise your muscles, burn more calories

Ever wonder why you see people in the gym doing the same cardio workouts, week after week, month after month, with no noticeable change to their bodies? Wouldn't you think that all that energy expenditure would always cause a steady weight loss as well as toned and defined muscles?

Think again. Your body is a such an efficient energy saver—harking back again to our cave-dwelling days, when food was scarce and no one knew when the next meal was arriving or how calorie dense it would be—that it prefers to minimize its energy expenditure. As a result, muscles quickly adapt to whatever they're being asked to do, so if you do the same workout time and again, you will be burning far fewer calories six months into your routine than you did the week you first started.

And don't forget that your brain isn't being stimulated by the same old routine, either. It says, in essence, *Hey, I can relax here.* And relax it does!

So you need to fight against your body's and your brain's inherent efficiency, and constantly and surprisingly switch things up every time you work out. Circuit training and doing an endless variety of similar yet different exercises with high repetitions and low weights keeps your brain sharp and your muscles getting a true workout instead of just going through the motions. The more they have to do something your brain perceives as new, the more blood will circulate, the more your heart rate will increase, and the more calories you'll burn.

Mixing it up is like recharging your own muscular batteries!

---

training for nonathletes. (Or, if you are already an athlete, it will condition you in a powerful new way.) And it also primes your brain to be able to flawlessly respond to any new commands you'll be giving it.

Stand Tall, Stand Strong: The Importance of Posture

I became obsessed with posture when I was leading a Walking for Fitness course run by the Central Park Conservancy in 2008. Dozens of people, of all different ages and sizes, mostly between fifty and eighty years of age, eagerly signed up, and off we went on a test walk so I could get an idea of how well they could move and what pace to set.

Well, the first thing I noticed was that they didn't look at me, or even ahead to where we were going. They looked down at the pavement. They were so afraid of stepping in a pothole or on uneven pavement that they threw their entire postural alignment out of whack.

You have to think about your eyes being focused in a straight line forward.

Right then and there, I decided to change the way they thought about walking, to teach them about correct posture.

Posture and Alignment

I'll bet you've seen and probably scoffed at photographs of young ladies walking around their deportment classes with books balanced on their heads. But that simple trick of balancing books on your skull is actually a terrific exercise in proper postural alignment, because it forces you to look straight ahead with your head up, eyes focused on the horizon. And that is the essence of good posture, since it properly aligns your neck with your spine. (For much more about how to walk, see chapter 11.)

Focusing your eyes on the horizon instead of on your feet automatically incorporates elements of balance into every walk. This is what sends signals, as you know, to and from your brain and the proprioceptive sensors of your sensory system. You're working your muscles so they hold your body straight up, which is a lot more work for them than if you slouched, and you're stimulating brain activity triggered by its need to keep you from toppling over.

Another incredibly important concept is that our bodies are designed to move forward. Every time you do that, however, you're working the muscles not just in the front of your body, but on the opposite side as well in an endless stream of contraction and stabilization, whether you realize it or not. (It helps to think of yourself as a three-dimensional creature.) So, for example, when you bend your knees the quadriceps in the front of your thighs contract, the hamstrings in the back of your thighs stabilize.

In order to walk with perfect postural alignment, all the muscles in the front and the back need to be equally flexible and strong. But here's the problem: as we walk, the muscles in the front of our bodies almost always tend to be stronger than the muscles in the back to compensate for the fact that we're almost always moving forward. You can test this yourself if you try to walk backward and realize how hard it is—not just because we need all our proprioceptive skill to do an unnatural movement, but because our back muscles are so much weaker.

Doing the Super Body, Super Brain exercises will give you so much core strength that you will no longer have to think about engaging and contracting your muscles when you walk: your body will do it for you automatically. I had my Central Park walkers do a few quick circuits before we got going. In only a few short weeks, their posture, speed, and fluidity of movement had all improved markedly.

Good posture isn't just about striding confidently with your eyes focused forward. It's especially necessary if you work at a desk job or spend a lot of time sitting at a desk. Few people have their workstations ergonomically designed, with keyboards and monitors placed so that they enhance strong posture rather than forcing you to slump or hunch over. When you sit improperly during the day, by the time you're ready to go home, your upper-body muscles have had to overcompensate so that you could get your work done. You'll be stiff and sore and tired, with a neck that's aching and a back that's twanging with discomfort.

Be sure to place the center of your computer monitor at eye level. You should not be looking down at it. (I fixed mine by placing it on a sturdy stack of large, thick books.) Do your utmost to do a quick five-minute stretch every hour. Also be aware of how you sit when you talk on the phone. Leaning to one side will throw your alignment off, too.

Breathe Deep

Who knows how to breathe properly? Yogis, opera singers, clarinet players—and babies. A baby comes out of the womb knowing how to breathe—watch an infant's belly move up and down with each correct breath—yet as we get older, our breathing shifts from instinctive belly breathing, using our diaphragm and abdominal muscles, to head breathing, either through our nose or mouth. Plus, most people do not use their full range of breath, as they breathe only into their midchest and neglect the lower and upper lungs.

Breathing correctly is a vital element of the Super Body, Super Brain routine. Using your diaphragm correctly allows you to bring much more oxygen not only into your lungs but to your entire body. If you think of your body as a machine, oxygen is the fuel that allows it to run. Wouldn't you rather fill up with premium fuel than cut-rate junk?

Best of all, oxygen is free, and maximizing its power not only is extremely easy but makes you feel great. Proper breathing is just like any other physical process. Don't take it for granted, and you can quickly become better at it with very little effort. Training yourself to breathe involves taking your lungs outside of their normal pat-

easy desk stretch

Try to remember to stretch your upper body at least once an hour. This can be done sitting or standing.

- Cup your hands behind your head, and then pull your elbows all the way back. Breathe deeply.

- When you feel a nice tension (not pain!) in the back of your shoulders, uncup your hands and stretch your arms gently up toward the ceiling. Hold for ten seconds.

- In the same position, look up at the ceiling while slightly moving your head backward and over to one side. Hold for ten seconds, and then repeat on the other side. It's a very simple movement that can do wonders for your neck.

terns of inhale/exhale and learning how to use your diaphragm rather than accessory muscles to take the deepest and most refreshing breath.

Conscious breathing usually slows down your heart rate and can instantly shift your focus away from whatever is upsetting you or engaging you. It's hard to yell at a selfish driver who just cut you off if you're concentrating on your breathing!

The children I work with love to be taught how to breathe. To them, it's just another game, since they don't have those self-critical little voices telling them that conscious breathing is for wimps. Together, we slowly breathe in and out, and I instantly see their eyes clear and their energy focus inward rather than outward. This helps calm them down after an energetic exercise session. It will give you a terrific sense of tranquillity after your workouts, too.

New York City yoga teacher (and one of my clients) Rebecca Victor-Hobert has shared her tips to help you breathe better and more deeply. She knows that proper breathing is so important because it:

- increases lung capacity and endurance
- helps maintain physical and mental focus during all types of activity
- gives you increased flexibility in your torso muscles
- can be used as a tool to raise or lower heart rate
- can be used to help you relax and/or meditate

Breathing Exercises

Each breath has three parts: inhalation, exhalation, and retention. You can do retention exercises on either the inhale or the exhale; it's more mentally challenging on the exhale.

Try to do these exercises whenever you have the time, the more the better, in a quiet place to focus. I suggest you do them at least two or three times each week.

1. Explore Diaphragmatic Breath

A. Lie on your back on the floor and then place one hand on your belly around the navel and the other hand on your chest.

B. Take a deep breath in through your nose. If only your chest rises, you are using mostly accessory muscles to breathe, not the full range of the diaphragm. If your belly rises, it's being efficiently activated. (In order to contract, the diaphragm pushes the organs of the abdomen down, allowing the lungs to inflate.)

2. Explore Lung Capacity

A. Lie on your back on the floor and then place your hands on either side of your torso around your lower ribs.

B. Inhale and exhale deeply.

C. Attempt to circumferentially expand your torso, from top to bottom, from side to side, and from back to front.

D. Flip over onto your belly and do the same. This time, feel your back open and expand as your belly releases into the floor. Try to create more space between each set of ribs in the back of your body. The front ribs are generally much more mobile and easily accessible than the back ribs; however, flexibility in the back ribs can be cultivated over time. Gaining access to the back body can even improve your posture over time!

3. Three-Part Breath

A. Lie down so that your abdominal muscles can relax rather than hold your torso upright. (After some practice, you can also do this exercise in a comfortable cross-legged position.) Place one hand on your navel and the other on your solar plexus region.

B. Breathe in through your nose, thinking only of inhaling into the hand on your navel, for a count of two.

C. Pause for one count. Direct the breath into the midchest (the hand on the solar plexus) for a count of two. Hold for one count.

D. Place one hand on the upper chest around your clavicle. Inhale there for two counts. Hold for one count.

E. Let it all out in one long, smooth exhalation.

Reps: 3–4

• Because your inhale occurs in three stages, make sure that you don't take in too much air in steps B and C.

• As you gain experience, you can increase the amount of time for both the inhalation and retention. For example, inhale for a count of four and pause for a count of two.

• If you are pregnant or have heart and/or blood pressure conditions, do this exercise without the pauses.

4. Reverse Inhalation and Exhalation via Rapid Breath

This breath focuses on an active exhalation with a passive inhalation. It is the opposite of a normal breathing pattern, which comprises an active inhalation and a passive exhalation. The goal of this exercise is to force air out of your lungs by rapidly contracting your abdominal muscles.

A. Sit in a comfortable cross-legged position. Your spine should be vertical and your head aligned with the base of your spine.

B. In order to understand the role of the abdominal muscles in this exercise, place one hand on your belly around your navel.

C. Initially, use the force of your hand to firmly press your belly back toward your spine while exhaling through your nose.

D. Release, and allow the inhalation to be almost passive.

E. Either remain with your hand on your belly to aid in the exhalation or try to do the same belly contraction/exhalation solely by using the belly muscles, not your hand.

F. Inhale a deep breath through your nose, and then exhale through your nose, making sure that you completely empty your lungs.

G. Inhale to a comfortable level and then begin a round of short, sharp exhalations through your nose, using the abdominal muscles as described in steps C, D, and E. You will make a sniffing sound.

Reps: 30 rounds (that is, 30 exhalations and inhalations)

• As you get better at this exercise, you can speed up the exhalations.

H. After the 30 rapid exhalations, slow them down.

I. Inhale completely and exhale fully, and then sip the air in to a comfortable level.

J. Contract your pelvic floor in and up. Then drop your chin to your chest and retain the breath for as long as feels comfortable.

K. When you need to release the breath, relax the pelvic floor, and then lift your chin back up.

Reps: 3 (steps F-K)

• Notice what comes up in the mind during the retention. Does your mind tell you to breathe before you really need to take a breath in?

• You can try this retention on both an in-breath, as described above, and an out-breath.

• As you gain experience with this exercise, try to increase the amount of time you hold the retention.

About Meditation

For me, meditation is an amazingly empowering tool that builds upon the techniques of conscious breathing for a more potent, calming self-awareness. I always incorporate meditation into my training sessions because I see how well it works, every time.

When you do a short, sweet meditation before you start exercising, it sets your intention and helps focus your mind on the task at hand. Becoming more mindful and acknowledging what you're about to do makes you more in tune with both your brain and your body. You can say whatever you like as long as it's positive and uncritical—such as these words provided by Sharon Salzberg, cofounder of the Insight Meditation Society: "I don't need to be impatient or judgmental to reach my goals" or "May I treat myself with kindness."

And when you do a short, sweet meditation at the end of your circuits, it slows down your breathing and helps you bring your heart rate gradually back down to normal, leaving you energized yet refreshed and relaxed. Acknowledge your hard work, even if you aren't particularly happy with what you did. (It's OK to say something like, "Even if I feel I blew it, I can always begin again. And I will.") It's the ideal way to give yourself a lovely sense of tranquillity after a workout, since you're flooded with endorphins and a marvelous sense of calm and accomplishment.

I have been very fortunate to have been tutored in the power of meditation by world-renowned Sharon Salzberg.

Sharon told me: "There is a common, mistaken idea that meditation is about stopping thoughts [it isn't—it involves developing a better relationship to our thoughts, not about becoming blank] and people feel that they could never do that, and so they will fail. But actually, meditation can be done by anyone looking for more clarity and centeredness in their life. All you need is a little time, compassion for yourself, and your breath.

"What is the minimum amount of time you need to [meditate] in order to see results? I think that consistency is more important than a length of time each day. If you can set aside twenty minutes every day or nearly every day, that is perfect. But if you only have five minutes a day, it is definitely worth doing. The results usually begin to manifest not in our formal sitting practice, but in life (which is where it really counts). You might notice that you start to get anxious in a meeting, but then remember to breathe. You might find yourself more able to let go of a spate of self-judgment, and more able to begin again when you've strayed from a chosen course of action. You might notice that a simple thing like drinking a cup of tea is more pleasant because you are more aware and in the moment with the experience."

Basic Meditation Instruction

Try your best to do this at a time and place where you will not be disturbed. This is your time for *you*. However, interruptions will happen. Don't let them upset you or throw you off balance. It might help to set an alarm so that you have a sense of when the session is done without having to check the time.

Sit in any position that's comfortable. A chair is fine, but do try to sit upright. You can also lie down and meditate. You can close your eyes or not, depending on how you feel most at ease. Feel free to change position if you need to, but try not to shift just out of restlessness.

Start by feeling your breath as it enters and leaves your nostrils. This is the normal, natural breath; do not try to make it deeper, or different. Rest your attention on the actual sensations of the breath. You may feel tingling, vibration, warmth, coolness; you don't have to name these, but feel them. If you like, you can use a very quiet mental note, such as "In . . . out," to help support awareness of your breathing.

If sounds or images or emotions or sensations other than the nostrils arise, let them flow on by. You don't need to fight them or follow after them . . . you're just breathing. It's like spotting a friend in a crowd: you don't have to shove aside everyone else, but your interest and your enthusiasm are going toward your friend. As in, "Oh, there's my friend. There's the breath."

If something arises that is strong enough to pull you away, or if you fall asleep, or if you get lost in a fantasy, don't worry about it. This is a moment to practice some compassion toward yourself, without harshness or self-condemnation. Let go of the distraction and simply begin again. Know that your mind will wander. Just notice where it went, and then gently bring it back to the breath— every time, over and over.

You will think and feel many things, both emotionally and physically, while you meditate. It is all OK. Just gently bring yourself back to the breath. Important insights may arise as well. Don't worry: you won't forget them.

Above all, have patience with and compassion for yourself. Each of us faces our own challenges in meditation, but the rewards are well worth it if we are kind to ourselves and keep on breathing!

PART TWO

SUPER BODY, SUPER BRAIN

Exercises

5

Basics Are Essential

B ecause the Super Body, Super Brain program is unique, this chapter will cover everything you need to know about the circuits you'll find in the ensuing chapters. You'll
soon see that these exercises will have the same powerful effect whether you're a professional athlete or a newbie to exercise.

Self-Diagnosis FITNESS QUIZ

Before beginning your program, take this simple quiz to assess your fitness level, balance,
coordination, strength, cardiovascular ability, flexibility, and cognitive skills. Not only will
it clearly show you how balance and coordination can actually be a brain-related "exercise,"
but it will direct you to the correct starting level of exercise.

Mark each answer with an *E* for Easy, *C* for Challenging, or *D* for Difficult.

BALANCE

- Raise both heels and raise your arms. Hold for ten seconds.   _____
- Do the same with your eyes closed.   _____

COORDINATION

■ Raise your opposite arm and leg for thirty seconds. ———

■ Do the same with one eye open. ———

■ Do the same with your eyes closed. ———

■ Walk forward, heel to toe, for ten steps and then backward
for ten steps. ———

STRENGTH

■ For lower-body strength, stand with your back against a wall
and with both knees bent at a ninety-degree angle, as if you were
sitting on a chair. Stay at that angle for forty-five seconds. ———

CARDIOVASCULAR

■ From a seated position, stand up, finishing on your toes,
and then sit down. This is one rep. Do two sets of twenty reps,
resting ten seconds between sets. Repeat the sequence. ———

FLEXIBILITY

■ From a standing position, cross one leg in front
of the other and touch your ankles. From that crossed
position, raise your arms above your head. ———

COGNITIVE SKILLS

■ Meditate or sit quietly with your thoughts for five minutes. ———

■ Were you able to tune out distractions and focus
on what you wanted to think about? ———

VISUALIZATION

■ Visualize yourself doing any exercises or movement
that you're used to doing, in perfect form. ———

LEARNING AND MEMORY

■ Read the headlines of your local newspaper for forty-five seconds.
Put the newspaper down, and then write down as many headlines as
you can remember. ———

SCORING

- If most of your answers are marked *D* (Difficult), start with no hand weights.
- If most of your answers are marked *C* (Challenging), start with no more than 3-pound hand weights.
- If most of your answers are marked *E* (Easy), use 3- to 7.5-pound weights.

What Are the Basics of Each Routine?

Even though each routine takes only about ten minutes, each one has been carefully designed to contain all these components, in a specific, balanced, progressive order:

- Mind-set/visualization
- Stretching
- Motor Skills—warm-up
- Motor Skills—cardio
- Motor Skills—cardio-strength
- Core Strength—obliques
- Proprioception/sensory
- Motor Skills—done on the floor
- Motor Skills—strength
- Stretching
- Meditation

What Equipment Do I Need?

You'll need only the following:

■ Hand weights

For beginners who've never used hand weights before, don't worry—you can start without them. As you progress, hold a soup can or a filled water bottle in each hand.

Since these are very precise and controlled movements, you'll know when you're ready to move up to regular hand weights.

I suggest that women purchase a set of hand weights (also called dumbbells) from 1 pound to 5 pounds, and men from 1 pound to 7.5 pounds. You can always hold two weights in each hand if you want a higher weight.

Even if you are an experienced weight lifter, you should start with only low-weight hand weights. You do not need heavier weights for faster results; in fact, using them will be counterproductive.

■ Exercise mat or carpet

All the exercises should be done on a padded surface. If you have carpeting or a well-secured area rug, you don't need a mat.

If you feel any discomfort in your knees when doing any of the floor exercises, you can place a pillow under them.

■ Timer

A kitchen timer can help you keep track of your time. You don't need to use it, though, until you've mastered all the exercises and no longer need to look at the photographs, since this will affect how long it takes you to do each circuit.

Exercise shoes

Believe it or not, some of my personal-training clients like to do their routines barefoot, but I think you have more stability and cushioning for your feet when you wear comfortable and supportive exercise shoes.

How Long Does It Take to Memorize These Exercises?

Again, results will vary. But you'll find that the more you do these exercises, the more quickly you'll master the more challenging levels, so that Level 4 will actually be much easier to learn and do than Level 1. That's because you will already have muscle memory as well as new neural networks.

How Often Should I Do These Exercises?

Even beginners should try to do these routines six times a week, once each day. These routines take only about ten min-

HOW OFTEN TO DO THE EXERCISES

SINGLE CIRCUIT: FOR THOSE WITH JUST 10 MINUTES

LEVEL	Week 1	Week 2	Week 3	Week 4
Monday	10	10	10	10
Tuesday	10	10	10	10
Wednesday	10	10	10	10
Thursday	10	10	10	10
Friday	10	10	10	10
Saturday	10	10	10	10
Sunday	rest	10	rest	10
Total minutes	60	70	60	70

MULTIPLE CIRCUITS: FOR THOSE WITH MORE THAN 10 MINUTES

LEVEL	Week 1	Week 2	Week 3	Week 4
Monday	10	2x10	10	2x10
Tuesday	2x10	10	2x10	10
Wednesday	10	2x10	10	10
Thursday	rest	rest	rest	10
Friday	10	10	2x10	2x10
Saturday	2x10	10	10	10
Sunday	rest	10	2x10	2x10
Total minutes	70	80	90	100

utes, yet will give you substantial physical and brain benefits

As you know already, according to the Mayo Clinic, doing three ten-minute sessions spread out during the day is even more beneficial than one thirty-minute session. The reason is that your total energy expenditure during multiple sessions is higher than the expenditure achieved during a single session per day. You'll also be stimulating your metabolism three times, not just once, so you'll burn slightly more calories when you regularly stoke your metabolic furnace.

It also might be a lot easier for you to find the odd ten minutes during the day than to find thirty solid minutes. This is what I often do; I'll work out first thing in the morning, again around lunchtime, and then when I get home at night. I find that the last session is the most important, because it helps me center myself at home after a long day at work.

Unless you are an advanced exerciser or professional athlete, you don't need to do more than three sessions each day.

How Long Should I Stay at Each Level?

You'll be at each level for at least four weeks, depending on your fitness level.

If you feel confident with all the exercises after two weeks at any level, you can then gradually increase the size of your hand weights while doing the same movements.

This gradual progression is based on the progressive-training techniques my Spanish basketball coaches used with my team-mates and me. The exercises we did during the preseason were never the same as those we did during the season itself, when we had to concentrate on performance. And the exercises we did in the postseason were primarily about conditioning and giving our bodies a rest from the intense levels of play. This helped us prevent injuries, stay focused on specific goals, and give different muscles different workouts, and it kept us from getting bored doing the same old exercises.

How Do I Know If I'm Doing Each Movement Properly?

Each movement is split into two sequences: when you start, and when you finish. You'll know if you're doing the movement in a proper, smooth, and coordinated way if, when you finish the movement, you can hold the position for two or three seconds. If you can't, don't worry; it just means you need a little bit more work on your balance and movement control. The more you do the exercises, the more these elements will improve.

When Will I See Results?

Everybody is different, and everybody responds differently to exercise. Some people tone up very quickly and show muscle definition in only a few weeks, while others need to be more patient. Obviously, though, if you do the exercise routine two or three times each day, you'll see results more quickly.

A guaranteed way to see faster results is to spend some time doing a nonimpact cardio routine several times a week. This can be doing something as simple as walking (see chapter 11 for more about walking for fitness). Or, if you go to a gym, I recommend no more than thirty-five to forty minutes on the elliptical machine, rowing machine, bicycle, or any combination; treadmills and stair-steppers are high impact. Add the Super Body, Super Brain routine *afterward,* since you'll be warmed up and the structure of the exercises makes them foolproof. Plus, you'll be working all the muscles in your body.

You can see results even if you're starting these exercises very slowly or after an injury. They'll help anyone, even those who are elderly or out of shape. We lose muscle volume and bone density when we age, contributing to poor posture and lack of neuromuscular efficiency. These exercises will *override* the usual aging process, so everyone will see a rapid improvement in how they stand, sit, and move.

Should I Rest Between Each Exercise and Each Circuit?

The program has been designed so that you do not need to rest between each exercise, but depending on your level, you should rest between each circuit.

When Do I Increase My Weights, and How Much Should I Add On?

You should very gradually increase your weights. Work out for at least two weeks per level with the starting weight, and only then should you advance up one weight level while remaining at the same exercise level. You'll go from no weight to one pound in each hand, then on to 2, 3, and 5, which will be enough for most exercisers; advanced levels can go up to 7.5, 8, 10, and 12 pounds.

When you're ready to move up to the next exercise level—from Level 1 to Level 2, perhaps—go back down to your initial starting weight at the previous level. Repeat the increase after two weeks.

So, for example, if you start with 3 pounds, after the initial sixteen weeks on the Super Body, Super Brain program you could have gradually increased your weights until you're up to 7.5 pounds—but only if you wanted to. (And at that point, you'll also be ready to integrate the different circuits.)

You'll know if the weights are too heavy if they distract you from doing the movements with perfect fluidity or if you feel out of breath really easily. Even after all the years I've spent doing these routines, I never use weights heavier than 15 pounds. It's much more important to concentrate on form than on weights; less can definitely be more!

Furthermore, lighter weights are better for those who prefer to get defined and toned faster, and who want to look long and lean. The heavier the weight, the more bulk it will add. So most women prefer to use weights in the 3- to 5-pound range, even after many months doing these exercises.

How Fast Should I Do the Circuits?

I've shown the recommended times—for beginners to athletes—at the beginning of each exercise chapter. How fast you do the circuits is entirely up to you, but here are some general guidelines:

Low Intensity: 2–1–1 Pattern. This means you do the first movement in two seconds, the second in one second, and then hold it for one second.

Medium Intensity: 1–1–1 Pattern. This means you do the first movement in one second, the second in one second, and then hold it for one second.

High Intensity: 0.5–0.5–0.5 Pattern. This means you do the first movement in half a second, the second in half a second, and then hold it for half a second.

Your body will tell you when it's ready for the next challenge. Be sure to listen to it! If you find the next level too difficult at first, drop back one level, keep at it for a few weeks, and then try again.

Don't ever compare yourself with anyone else. This isn't a race. Your only competition is with yourself. Your goal is to improve your time, little by little.

Every time you do the routine, you're a winner!

Does It Matter Which Side I Start On?

I'm left-handed, so I always start on my left side. I've been very specific about which side to start on, so follow the instructions carefully. Every circuit is perfectly balanced between right and left.

Starting on the opposite of your dominant side always adds another challeng-

ing element to your routine. When you are ready to move on to more advanced levels, you can switch up the starting side to keep the routines even more fresh.

Why Can't I Look at My Legs or Feet When I'm Doing These Exercises?

Since all the movements are based on controlled imbalance, you want to enable your muscles and postural alignment to be perfectly engaged. Otherwise, you won't be able to do the exercises properly.

Which is why it's so important for your back to remain straight, when indicated, and for your eyes to always be fixed on a point either straight ahead (when you're standing) or on the ceiling (when you're lying on your back). Keeping your eyes fixed on a specific point will keep your neck perfectly positioned, which is necessary for your posture to be correctly aligned.

In addition, when your eyes are fixed on a point in the distance, you will be less likely to swing your head or lose your balance—neither of which you want to do!

I'm Used to Exercising with Music—Can I Use It for These Routines?

Music can be a great motivator when you're doing cardiovascular exercise and you want to keep your heart rate up and steady. But these exercises are different: you'll be concentrating so powerfully that you might find that the music you're used to becomes a distraction. So I don't recommend that beginners do these routines with any music to trick their brains into not focusing on the task at hand.

Once you've mastered all the movements, however, feel free to add music if it helps or pleases you, as long as it doesn't interfere with the precision of your routines.

What If I'm Already an Experienced Athlete?

No matter how accomplished an athlete you are, everyone needs to start at Level 1, with the exercises in chapter 5. You'll pick up the routines more quickly than a beginner would, and you'll be able to work with a higher amount of weights and with less resting time between circuits. But you'll still need to concentrate on your intensity and on performing the movements perfectly.

What About Pain?

Pain is like a fever—a symptom that something is wrong. It is absolutely never OK to disregard pain or think you can work around it and it will somehow magically disappear. I always tell my clients to listen to their bodies—and not ignore what they're hearing! As an athlete who has often, and stupidly, gritted my teeth to get through pain, I know how counterproductive if not downright dangerous it is to ignore your body's signals that something is wrong.

Super Body, Super Brain exercises should never hurt. If, however, you're sore or stressed or not paying attention, you may feel some discomfort while or after doing a specific movement. This often happens to those who progress on to heavier weights before they're actually strong enough to do so.

If you feel little pings or twitches or any discomfort whatsoever, crank it down a notch. Do not move up a level or try to increase any of the variables until you are stronger and can seamlessly execute every movement, easily and with perfect form. As you know, this is not a race, and the more gently you ease into exercising, the more satisfying your progress will be.

I Love My Cardio Exercise— Do I Have to Change My Routine?

Cardiovascular exercise has important health benefits, as you know. It strengthens your heart, improves your circulation, and is a great stress reliever. As you can see in the sidebar with my own routine, I do no more than thirty-five minutes of nonimpact cardio exercise at least twice a week in addition to my thrice-daily Super Body, Super Brain circuits.

Adding a fast and effective strength-training workout together with no-impact exercises will enhance any cardio routine. In fact, I devised this program partly in response to seeing so many people exercising in the gym, getting off the machines after running for forty-five minutes, and then not having a clue as to what to do with the hand weights or weight machines. Then they either did nothing—or did a whole lot of exercises wrong, which not only was counterproductive but could have easily led to some serious injuries.

ward's story

"I'm forty-four and have been one of Michael's clients for several years. His workouts have been hugely beneficial for me as a surfer.

"Surfing is the kind of sport where you have to break down what you're really doing. Most people think the hard work is getting up on the board and dealing with the waves, but the really tough stuff and the endurance component is when you're paddling through big surf to get out to the waves. So it's really important to have upper-body strength as well as core strength if you want to surf well. You spend a lot of time banana'd on the board, where your legs and spine are flat and, in what's like an extended plank position, where you need to elevate your shoulders, so you can see over the waves.

"In addition, there's a critical transition in the water, where you're flat while you're paddling, but then you suddenly have to jump up and stand on the board. This necessitates an extreme energy burst—but what's tricky at the same time is that you get this huge adrenaline rush, but then you immediately have to calm yourself so that you remain relaxed and fluid enough to stay balanced on the board. If you're too rigid, you'll always fall.

"So, for me, Michael's workout is so effective because it has enabled me to strengthen all my muscles as well as my reflexes, so I can pop up to the surfing position and find my balance immediately. Michael's exercises always have you focused on doing at least two different movements simultaneously, so that's the perfect training for surfing. I now have the fluidity of movement as well as a keen sense of balance thanks to his strengthening my stabilizing muscles. As a result, my skill level as a surfer has gone up exponentially.

"The Super Body, Super Brain exercises have also improved my balance tremendously for my golf game. Not just my physical coordination—because golf is also a mental game. I now have additional strength and flexibility, so I don't have to swing as hard. I can do a three-quarter swing with the same power and much more accuracy.

"I've also noticed that my reflexes have sharpened in little ways. If I'm fumbling around in the medicine cabinet and knock a bottle of aspirin over, I can catch it in a flash. It's not something I have to think about anymore—this instinctiveness of movement. I'm more highly tuned, so I know there's definitely something going on mentally. It's extremely exhilarating."

In addition, these routines will complement regular sports activities, easing the strain on your joints and helping you play the sport longer and at a higher level. In fact, those who like to do certain sports will find that their workouts should show considerable improvement once they incorporate these routines into their regular sessions. The reason is that once you're able to multitask, improve your balance and coordination, and drastically strengthen your core muscles and upper-body strength, all movements that you do will be smoother, stronger, and more pre-

cise. This will be especially noticeable if you play a sport involving hand-eye coordination (tennis, baseball, hockey), multitasking (basketball, soccer, football), or running (both sprinting and long distance).

If I Need to Take Time Off from Doing Any Exercise, What Level Should I Go To When I Start Exercising Again?

Always go back to the level you started with. You should find it quickly coming

MY OWN ROUTINE

After doing these exercises for so long, I am now in Level 7, which is a combination of exercises from Level 1 + Level 3 + Level 4. I vary my circuits and combine them several times a week with no more than 35 minutes of non-impact cardio exercise, as you'll see in this chart. My initial starting weight is 12 pounds, and if I feel I need an upgrade I always wait at least 2 weeks at the 12-pound level before moving up to 15 pounds, which is the highest weight level I will ever need to use.

LEVEL	Week 1	Week 2	Week 3	Week 4
Monday	10	35'+10	10	35'+10
Tuesday	2 x 10	2x10	35'+10	2x10
Wednesday	35'+10	35'+10	2x10	35'+10
Thursday	rest	10	rest	3x10
Friday	10	2x10	2x10	2x10
Saturday	2x10	10	3x10	2x10
Sunday	35'+10	rest	35'+10	rest
Total	150	150	170	180

back to you, and if so, you can perhaps add a slightly higher level of weights. Once you feel completely comfortable with the routine, you can quickly move forward to the level you'd reached when you took the break.

How Do I Know When I'm Ready for the Next Level?

Before you move on to the next level, you'll need to master all the different movements in each exercise and have them memorized so you don't need to refer to the photographs in this book any longer.

There are many different elements to master, too. You'll find yourself transitioning from hesitant to smooth, from slower to faster, from no weights to heavier weights. I recommend that you do each exercise for two weeks before adding another element. So, for example, you can do the circuits more quickly, and when you're comfortable with that, you can increase your weights.

Once you've mastered all the routines in the next four chapters, you'll find all the information you need about moving on to the next levels in chapter 9.

Mental Preparation Before You Exercise

When I used to play semiprofessional basketball in Spain, I always followed a very specific pregame mental warm-up that was as important as my physical warm-up.

First I ran through a mental checklist to reinforce my readiness to play; to concentrate with precision, intensity, and awareness; and to be ready to have that mental energy available when I was called onto the court. After a few minutes of this tune-up, I would do a few minutes of deep breathing, which would send a signal to my sensory system that I was primed for play. My fingers would actually start moving as if I were holding the ball and ready to dribble and shoot.

Finding that sweet spot of mental preparation prior to exercise (or before undertaking any task) is often called entering the zone. I spoke to sports psychologist Patrick Cohn, Ph.D., founder of Peak Performance Sports, about this, and he told me that the zone is simply a mental state of total involvement in the present moment. "I like the word *immersed*," he told me, "as it indicates that you lose yourself—or your sense of self—when you perform."

You can do this kind of mental prep work, too. It means you'll be tuning out all other thoughts, fear, or worries and concentrating solely on the deeply satisfying physical and mental challenge of the exercise routine you're about to do. Visualize yourself doing the exercises with smooth confidence and strength—and you'll be able to create the ideal, powerful mental energy to enhance your workout.

You should also try to do a very brief meditation session before each exercise session, which will help you set an intention. Take a minute or so to do some deep breathing, and tell yourself, "I don't need to be impatient or judgmental to reach my goals." Or "May I treat myself with kindness." Or "Even if I feel like I blew it last time, I can always begin again." Reinforcing your strengths and your power will always automatically improve your exercise abilities.

Basic Exercises

This list contains the most common exercises used in every chapter. Some of them, like the Crunch, might not be what you're used to doing, because they are unique to this book. So familiarize yourself with these movements before your start your circuit.

Bicep Curl

❏ Pick up your hand weights and hold them firmly, arms straight and palms facing forward.

❏ Bend your elbows and bring your arms up to shoulder height. You will feel the contraction of the biceps muscle in the front of your upper arm.

❏ Return to the starting position. This is one rep.

Be sure to keep your elbow very slightly bent; your arm should not be totally straight or rigid.

Chest Press

❏ Lie flat on your back, head back, eyes focused on the ceiling.

❏ Holding the weights, spread your arms out to the sides, perpendicular to your body, at shoulder height. Then bend your elbows so that your arms are bent at a ninety-degree angle, palms facing forward. Your elbows should be aligned with your shoulders.

❏ Straighten your arms and extend them up. Keep them shoulder width apart.

❏ Return to the starting position. This is one rep.

Half Push-up

- ❑ Get down on the floor on your hands and knees, arms slightly more than shoulder width apart. Extend your left leg straight back, no higher than hip height.
- ❑ Bend your elbows slightly, and move your upper body halfway down to the floor. Keep your back leg extended out. Do not look at the floor; keep your eyes focused straight ahead.
- ❑ Return to the starting position. This is one rep.

Do not go all the way down to the floor. This is not a full push-up. Your elbows should be bent at no more than a ninety-degree angle.

The movement is very slightly forward, almost diagonal. You don't want to go straight up and down.

Semi-Lunge

- ❑ Stand tall, arms by your sides. Take two steps back with your left leg. Keep this leg straight, with your heel slightly off the floor. Bend your right knee slightly. Your weight is evenly distributed over both legs.
- ❑ Bend your right knee slightly; then push off with the toes of your left leg and bring your left knee up at a ninety-degree angle, toes pointing down.
- ❑ Return to the starting position. This is one rep.

Keep the heel of your back leg off the ground at all times.

Don't raise your knee higher than hip height.

Keep your back straight at all times or your weight will be unevenly distributed. This is a constant, smooth movement.

Do not look down; keep your eyes focused forward at all times.

Semi-Squat Plié / Heel Raise

- ❑ Stand up and place your legs comfortably more than shoulder width apart, knees bent slightly, with your feet pointing outward. You are in a turned-out position.
- ❑ Bend your knees slightly and lower your body, then straighten your knees back to the starting position. Finish by raising your heels slightly off the floor.
- ❑ Return to the starting position. This is one rep.

Never raise your heels more than an inch or two off the floor.

Shoulder Lateral Raise

❑ Stand tall, holding the weights, with your arms loosely at your sides, palms facing in. Keep your elbows slightly bent.

❑ Raise your arms out to the sides, to no more than shoulder height.

❑ Return to the starting position. This is one rep.

Triceps Extension—Lying Down

❑ Lie flat on your back, holding the weights, with your elbows bent and pointing upward, and your hands brought toward your forehead.

❑ Straighten your arms up toward the ceiling.

❑ Return to the starting position. This is one rep.

Triceps Extension—Standing

❑ Stand tall, holding the weights, with your elbows bent and back slightly and your hands at waist level, palms facing each other.

❑ Straighten your arms back behind you.

❑ Return to the starting position. This is one rep.

This is a smooth and small movement. Do not swing your arms back.

Keep your eyes focused straight ahead. Do not move your upper body forward or backward.

Upper Back Extension

❑ Standing, holding the weights, and with your arms extended at shoulder height, bend your elbows up at a ninety-degree angle, palms facing forward.

❑ Extend your arms straight up to the ceiling.

❑ Return to the starting position. This is one rep.

Your arms are moving up into a vertical position. Do not move them forward.

6

Level 1: The Owl

WOMEN

IF YOU ARE A BEGINNER

- Hand weights: 0–3 pounds
- Rest between circuits: 30–45 seconds
- Intensity: low-medium
- Approximate time per circuit: 3:30–4:30
- Approximate time per 3 circuits: 11:00–15:45

IF YOU ARE INTERMEDIATE

- Hand weights: 3–5 pounds
- Rest between circuits: 15–30 seconds
- Intensity: medium
- Approximate time per circuit: 3:00–3:30
- Approximate time per 3 circuits: 9:45–11:00

IF YOU ARE ADVANCED

- Hand weights: 5–7.5 pounds
- Rest between circuits: 5–15 seconds
- Intensity: medium-high
- Approximate time per circuit: 2:30–3:00
- Approximate time per 3 circuits: 7:45–9:45

If You Are an Athlete / Professional Player

- Hand weights: 7.5+ pounds
- Rest between circuits: none
- Intensity: high
- Approximate time per circuit: 2:00–2:30
- Approximate time per 3 circuits: 6:00–7:30

MEN

If You Are a Beginner

- Hand weights: 0–3 pounds
- Rest between circuits: 30–45 seconds
- Intensity: low-medium
- Approximate time per circuit: 3:30–4:30
- Approximate time per 3 circuits: 11:00–15:45

If You Are Intermediate

- Hand weights: 5–7.5 pounds
- Rest between circuits: 15–30 seconds
- Intensity: medium
- Approximate time per circuit: 3:00–3:30
- Approximate time per 3 circuits: 9:45–11:00

If You Are Advanced

- Hand weights: 7.5–10 pounds
- Rest between circuits: 5–15 seconds
- Intensity: medium-high
- Approximate time per circuit: 2:30–3:00
- Approximate time per 3 circuits: 7:45–9:45

If You Are an Athlete / Professional Player

- Hand weights: 10–12+ pounds
- Rest between circuits: none
- Intensity: high
- Approximate time per circuit: 2:00–2:30
- Approximate time per 3 circuits: 6:00–7:30

WOMEN and MEN

■ Follow the directions. Sometimes you'll start with your right leg and arm, sometimes with your left. All the circuits have been deliberately designed so that both sides of your body are worked out equally.

■ After two weeks of regular exercising, don't forget to gradually increase the amount of your hand weights. Never upgrade by more than 2 to 2.5 pounds. For example, if you start with 1-pound weights, your next weight can be 2 to 3 pounds; if you start with 3 pounds, your next weight will be 5 pounds.

■ It will take you a few days to master each circuit. Aim to reduce the time it takes you to do each circuit from the second week on.

■ For those who already have a regular cardiovascular routine, I prefer to add these Super Body, Super Brain circuits after you've finished your cardio.

Level 1: THE OWL

STEP 1: MIND-SET

Visualize the exercises for thirty seconds before you start, just as a professional athlete would—with concentration, intensity, precision, and proper form. Say, "I am going to do my best. I know I can do it." Breathe deeply.

STEP 2: ALWAYS STRETCH BEFORE YOU START

Stretching not only loosens you up but sends a signal to your brain that you're ready to work out.

Standing tall and straight, cross your left foot over your right foot.

With your arms straight, bend at the waist and drop your upper body down to touch your knees, ankles, or toes. If you are already used to stretching, do not bend your knees; if it's more comfortable, you can bend your knees slightly to avoid locking the joint. You should feel the stretch in the back of your legs.

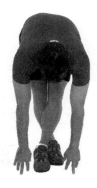

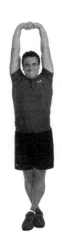

Hold this position for ten seconds. Then, without uncrossing your feet, raise your arms as high as you comfortably can. Look straight ahead and breathe deeply.

Switch feet, crossing your right foot over your left, and repeat the stretch.

STEP 3: **ENERGY BOOSTER: CLAP + BALANCE**

You can do this exercise whenever you feel sluggish during the day, too.

From a semi-squat-plié position, with your arms down at your sides, clap between your legs.

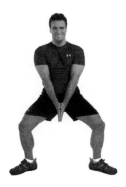

Stand up and then raise your heels while simultaneously raising your arms to clap overhead. Don't forget to smile!

Reps: 10

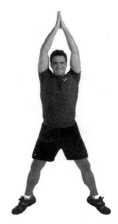

Every count should be coordinated with a loud voice. You can count from one to ten or shout out positive ideas like "Let's do it," "We can do it," and "Come on."

Do your clapping with as much speed as possible.

STEP 4: EXERCISE CIRCUITS

1. Opposite Arm and Leg Raise

Stand tall, with your feet close together, arms at your sides.

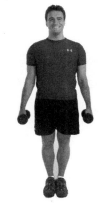

Raise your right arm above your head while simultaneously bending your left knee up at a ninety-degree angle, foot parallel to the floor.

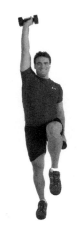

Repeat on the opposite side. This is one rep.

Reps: 12

This Exercise Is Good for:

Brain: balance, coordination, opposite arm and leg movement, posture alignment

Body: core strength; front thighs, glutes, shoulders

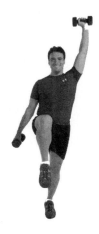

2. Leg Kick with Biceps Curl / Step Back and Forth

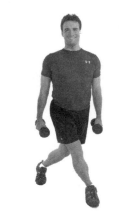

Stand tall, with your feet shoulder width apart, arms down at your sides. Cross your left leg slightly behind your right.

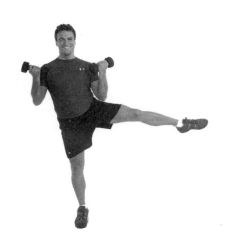

Kick your left leg out to the side while simultaneously doing biceps curls with both arms.

Change legs, and repeat on the other side. This is one rep.

Reps: 10

Ideally, these steps should be performed as quickly as possible, without losing the pattern. If you miss a step here and there, you're going too fast.

This Exercise Is Good for:

Brain: balance, coordination, footwork, speed, timing

Body: core strength; calves, front thighs, glutes, shoulders

3. Semi-Squat Plié with Shoulder Raise

Stand in the semi-squat-plié position, arms down between your knees, palms facing each other.

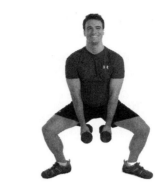

Standing tall, raise your heels slightly off the floor while simultaneously extending your arms straight out to the sides. This is one rep.

Reps: 8

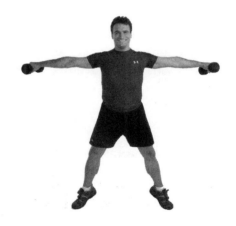

Be sure to keep your weight shifted back; you do not want to place your body forward over your knees. Your back should remain as straight as possible.

Do not raise your arms higher than your shoulders.

This Exercise Is Good for:

Brain: balance, coordination, multitasking limb movements, posture alignment, timing

Body: core strength; back, front, and inner thighs; calves, chest, glutes, shoulders

4. Semi-Squat Plié with Biceps Curl

Stand in the semi-squat-plié position, arms down in front of your thighs, palms facing out.

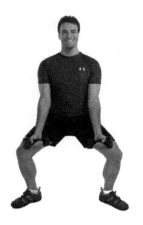

Standing tall, raise your heels slightly off the floor while simultaneously doing a biceps curls with both arms. This is one rep.

Reps: 8

Keep your arms as close in to your sides as possible. Your upper arms will barely move as you flex.

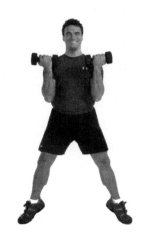

This Exercise Is Good for:

Brain: balance, coordination, multitasking limb movements, posture alignment, timing

Body: core strength; biceps, front thighs, glutes, shoulders, upper back

5. Semi-Squat Plié with Upper Back Extension

Stand in the squat-plié position, and then bend your arms up at a ninety-degree angle on both sides of your head.

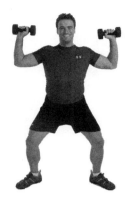

Standing tall, raise your heels slightly off the floor while simultaneously straightening your arms up toward the ceiling. This is one rep.

Reps: 8

This Exercise Is Good for:

Brain: balance, coordination, multitasking limb movements, posture alignment, timing

Body: core strength; front thighs, glutes, shoulders, upper back

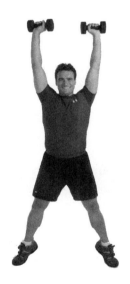

6. Semi-Squat Plié with Triceps Extension

Stand in the semi-squat-plié position, bending your elbows behind you at a ninety-degree angle, palms facing each other at your sides.

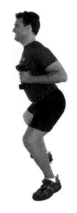

Standing tall, raise your heels slightly off the floor while simultaneously keeping your elbows stable and extending your arms back. This is one rep.

Reps: 8

Keep your back straight at all times. You do not want to swing the weights or pull them too far back; the motion backward should be smooth and should feel comfortable.

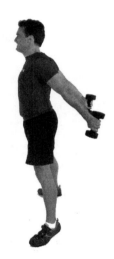

This Exercise Is Good for:

Brain: balance, coordination, multitasking limb movements, posture alignment, timing

Body: core strength; front thighs, glutes, shoulders, triceps, upper back

7. Semi-Squat Plié with Cross Jab

Stand in the semi-squat-plié position and then raise your heels slightly off the floor, arms raised to slightly below shoulder height, elbows bent at a ninety-degree angle.

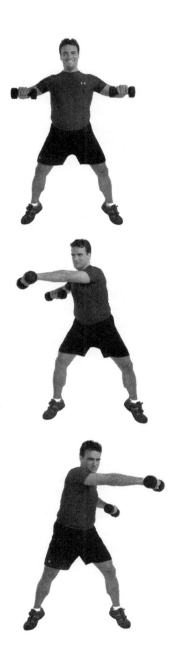

Extend your left arm across and forward to the right while twisting your waist to the left. Do not move your hips.

Repeat with the right arm. This is one rep.

Reps: 10

Make sure you are perfectly balanced, with your heels raised, during the entire exercise.

Do not raise your heels any higher than two inches off the floor or you might lose your balance.

Because most of the movement comes from your oblique abdominal muscles, you do not want to engage your hips at all.

This Exercise Is Good for:

Brain: controlled imbalance, coordination, multitasking movements (lower body is balancing while upper body is moving)

Body: core strength; back, front, and inner thighs; calves, chest, glutes, oblique abdominals, shoulders

8. Eyes Closed—Front Row

In the semi-squat-plié position, raise your heels slightly off the floor and then extend your arms straight out, keeping your hands at waist level and pointing toward the floor. Close your eyes.

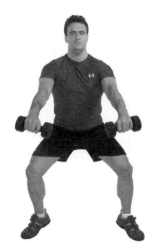

Bend your elbows and pull your arms in toward your body in a rowing motion. This is one rep.

Reps: 8

When you pull your arms back, keep your elbows away from your body.

Make sure to keep your eyes closed during the entire exercise.

When your eyes are closed, your brain and body are missing their regular cues and have to work much harder.

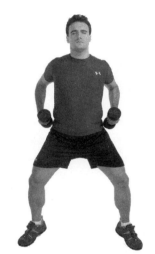

This Exercise Is Good for:

Brain: balance, coordination, posture alignment

Body: core strength; back and front thighs, biceps, calves, chest, glutes, middle back, shoulders

9. Opposite Arm and Leg Extension—

Get down on your hands and knees on the floor, hands shoulder width apart, with your back straight.

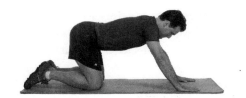

Simultaneously extend your left arm and your right leg.

Repeat on the other side. This is one rep.

Reps: 5

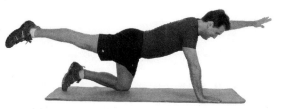

Do not raise your arm any higher than your shoulders.

Do not raise your leg any higher than your hips.

This Exercise Is Good for:

Brain: balance, coordination, multitasking limb movements, posture alignment

Body: core strength; back and front thighs, glutes, shoulders, upper back

10a. Straight Leg Raise—Floor

Get down on your hands and knees, and then extend your left leg horizontally behind you to below hip height. Point your toes to the floor so that your foot is at a ninety-degree angle to your leg.

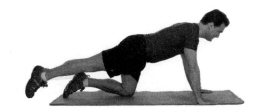

Raise your leg straight up no higher than hip height. This is one rep.

Reps: 8

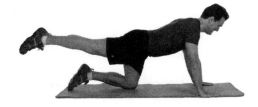

10b. Straight Leg Raise with Push-up—Floor

With your leg still up and extended, bend your upper body down into a half-push-up.

Repeat the entire sequence on your right side.

Reps: 6

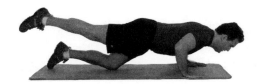

When you're doing the push-up, do not go down farther than a ninety-degree angle with your elbows. You don't need to do a full push-up.

This Exercise Is Good for:

Brain: balance, coordination, posture alignment, timing

Body: core strength; back thighs, chest, glutes, shoulders, triceps

11. Open-Leg Chest Press—Floor

Lie on your back with your legs up and your feet pointing toward the ceiling, shoulders and upper arms flat on the floor, elbows bent up at a ninety-degree angle, palms facing forward.

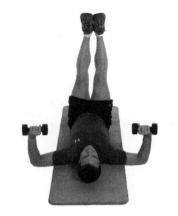

Open your legs while simultaneously extending your arms straight up, slightly more than shoulder width apart. This is one rep.

Reps: 8

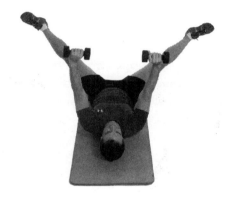

This Exercise Is Good for:

Brain: coordination, multitasking limb movements, timing

Body: abdominals, chest, front and inner thighs, glutes, shoulders, triceps

12. Bent-Leg Sit-up with Chest Press

Lie on your back with your knees bent at a ninety-degree angle with both legs off the floor, shoulders and upper arms flat on the floor, elbows bent up at a ninety-degree angle, palms facing forward. Keep your head flat on the floor.

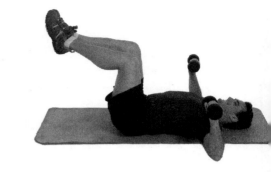

Lift your upper body off the floor while simultaneously raising your arms straight up, no more than shoulder width apart. This is one rep.

Reps: 8

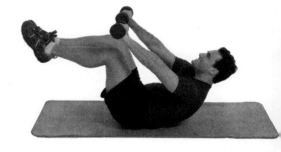

Do not look forward. Keep your eyes focused on the ceiling at all times.

If you feel a pull in your neck while lifting your upper body, you are not yet strong enough to raise yourself off the floor. Keep your head on the ground at all times until your core muscles become stronger.

This Exercise Is Good for:

Brain: coordination

Body: abdominals, chest, front and inner thighs, glutes, shoulders, triceps

13. Pelvic Raise with Chest Press

Lie on your back with your knees bent up at a ninety-degree angle, feet flat on the floor, shoulders and upper arms flat on the floor with elbows bent up at a ninety-degree angle, palms facing forward. Keep your head flat on the floor.

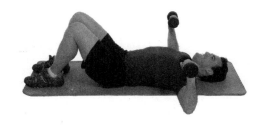

Lift your pelvis up as far as is comfortable while simultaneously raising your arms up, no more than shoulder width apart. This is one rep.

Reps: 8

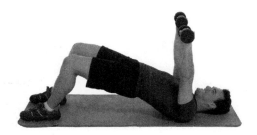

This Exercise Is Good for:

Brain: coordination, multitasking limb movements, timing

Body: abdominals, chest, front and inner thighs, glutes, shoulders, triceps

After you have done all the exercises, you will have finished one complete circuit.

Rest for zero to forty-five seconds, depending on your level, and then repeat the circuit two more times.

At the end of the third set, finish with a quick meditation cooldown. Ideally, you should aim for two to five minutes of meditation, but if you don't have time, even one minute will be extremely beneficial. Simply close your eyes, breathe deeply, congratulate yourself on the powerful work you have just done, and appreciate your strength and commitment. (Never judge yourself or be hard on yourself if you missed a movement or your circuit took longer than expected.) Then, mentally prepare yourself for the rest of your day.

7

Level 2: The Hawk

WOMEN

IF YOU ARE A BEGINNER

- Hand weights: 0–3 pounds
- Rest between circuits: 30–45 seconds
- Intensity: low-medium
- Approximate time per circuit: 3:30–4:30
- Approximate time per 3 circuits: 11:00–15:45

IF YOU ARE INTERMEDIATE

- Hand weights: 3–5 pounds
- Rest between circuits: 15–30 seconds
- Intensity: medium
- Approximate time per circuit: 3:00–3:30
- Approximate time per 3 circuits: 9:45–11:00

IF YOU ARE ADVANCED

- Hand weights: 5–7.5 pounds
- Rest between circuits: 5–15 seconds
- Intensity: medium-high
- Approximate time per circuit: 2:30–3:00
- Approximate time per 3 circuits: 7:45–9:45

If You Are an Athlete / Professional Player

- Hand weights: 7.5+ pounds
- Rest between circuits: none
- Intensity: high
- Approximate time per circuit: 2:00–2:30
- Approximate time per 3 circuits: 6:00–7:30

MEN

If You Are a Beginner

- Hand weights: 0–3 pounds
- Rest between circuits: 30–45 seconds
- Intensity: low-medium
- Approximate time per circuit: 3:30–4:30
- Approximate time per 3 circuits: 11:00–15:45

If You Are Intermediate

- Hand weights: 5–7.5 pounds
- Rest between circuits: 15–30 seconds
- Intensity: medium
- Approximate time per circuit: 3:00–3:30
- Approximate time per 3 circuits: 9:45–11:00

If You Are Advanced

- Hand weights: 7.5–10 pounds
- Rest between circuits: 5–15 seconds
- Intensity: medium-high
- Approximate time per circuit: 2:30–3:00
- Approximate time per 3 circuits: 7:45–9:45

If You Are an Athlete / Professional Player

- Hand weights: 10–12+ pounds
- Rest between circuits: none
- Intensity: high
- Approximate time per circuit: 2:00–2:30
- Approximate time per 3 circuits: 6:00–7:30

WOMEN and MEN

■ Follow the directions. Sometimes you'll start with your right leg and arm, sometimes with your left. All the circuits have been deliberately designed so that both sides of your body are worked out equally.

■ After two weeks of regular exercising, don't forget to gradually increase the amount of your hand weights. Never upgrade by more than 2 to 2.5 pounds. For example, if you start with 1-pound weights, your next weight can be 2 two 3 pounds; if you start with 3 pounds, your next weight will be 5 pounds.

■ It will take you a few days to master each circuit. Aim to reduce the time it takes you to do each circuit from the second week on.

■ For those who already have a regular cardiovascular routine, I prefer to add these Super Body, Super Brain circuits after you've finished your cardio.

Level 2: THE HAWK

Step 1: MIND-SET

Visualize the exercises for thirty seconds before you start, just as a professional athlete would—with concentration, intensity, precision, and proper form. Say, "I am going to do my best. I know I can do it." Breathe deeply.

Step 2: ALWAYS STRETCH BEFORE YOU START

Stretching not only loosens you up but sends a signal to your brain that you're ready to work out.

Standing tall and straight, cross your left foot over your right foot.

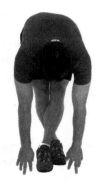

With your arms straight, **bend at the waist** and drop your upper body down to touch your knees, ankles, or toes. If you are already used to stretching, do not bend your knees; if it's more comfortable, you can bend your knees slightly to avoid locking the joint. You should feel the stretch in the back of your legs.

Hold this position for ten seconds. Then, without uncrossing your feet, raise your arms as high as you comfortably can. Look up toward the ceiling and breathe deeply.

Switch feet, crossing your right foot over your left, and repeat the stretch.

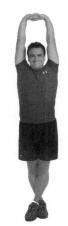

STEP 3: **ENERGY BOOSTER: CLAP + BALANCE**

You can do this exercise whenever you feel sluggish during the day, too.

From a semi-squat-plié position, with your arms down at your sides, clap between your legs.

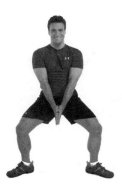

Stand up and then raise your heels while simultaneously raising your arms to clap overhead. Don't forget to smile!

Reps: 10

Every count should be coordinated with a loud voice. You can count from one to ten or shout out positive ideas like "Let's do it," "We can do it," and "Come on."

Do your clapping with as much speed as possible.

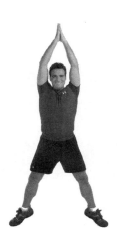

Step 4: EXERCISE CIRCUITS

1. Opposite Triceps Extensions and Leg Rais

Stand tall, with your feet close together, arms bent at your elbows.

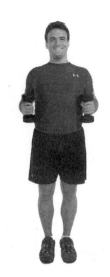

Hold the weights with both arms bent at the waist and then straighten your left arm behind you while simultaneously bending your right knee up at a ninety-degree angle, foot parallel to the floor.

Repeat on the opposite side. This is one rep.

Reps: 15

Be sure not to lean forward.

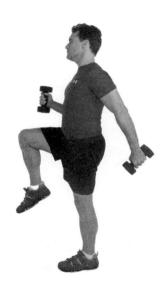

This Exercise Is Good for:

Brain: balance, coordination, opposite arm and leg movement, posture alignment

Body: core strength; front thighs, glutes, shoulders

2a. Leg Kick with Triceps Extension / Tapping

Stand tall, with your feet shoulder width apart, arms bent at your sides. Cross your left leg slightly behind your right.

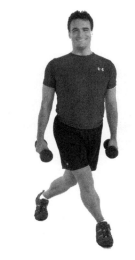

Kick your left leg out to the side while simultaneously extending both arms backward. This is one rep.

Reps: 10

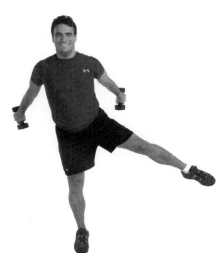

Keep your back straight at all times.

Beginners should feel comfortably balanced when they cross their legs behind; you don't want to lose your balance. The more advanced you are, the more you can extend the crossing action behind your leg.

Your hips should always be facing front. If they aren't, it means you're crossing too far and your balance will be out of whack.

2b. Leg Kick / Tapping

Stand tall, with your feet shoulder width apart, arms bent at your sides. With your toes pointed outward, slightly raise one foot and then quickly follow it with the other foot, like you're tapping your feet.

Change legs and repeat exercise 2a with the other leg.

Reps: 10

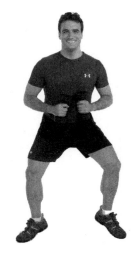

Think of the foot shift as almost a tapping movement, as if you were a basketball player defending your position.

Ideally, these steps should be performed as quickly as possible without losing the pattern. If you miss a step here and there, you're going too fast.

When doing exercise 2b, make sure you always alternate left and right feet when starting the exercise.

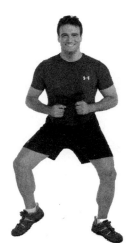

This Exercise Is Good for:

Brain: balance, coordination, footwork, speed, timing

Body: core strength; calves, front and inner thighs, glutes, shoulders

3. Semi-Lunge with Shoulder Raise

Stand tall, in the semi-lunge position, arms down comfortably between your hips and knees, palms facing each other.

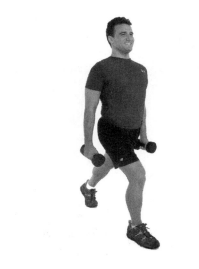

Raise your left leg by pushing it with your toes, until your left thigh is parallel to the floor while simultaneously extending your arms straight out to the sides. This is one rep.

Reps: 8

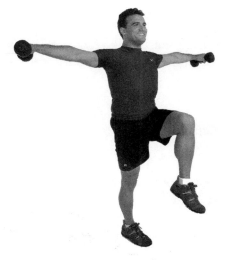

Be sure to keep your weight shifted back; you do not want to place your body forward over your knees. Your back should remain as straight as possible.

Do not raise your arms higher than shown in the photograph.

This Exercise Is Good for:

Brain: balance, coordination, multitasking limb movements, posture alignment, timing

Body: core strength; ankles; back, front, and inner thighs; calves, chest, glutes, knees, shoulders

4. Semi-Lunge with Biceps Curl

Stand in the semi-lunge position, arms down comfortably between your hips and knees, palms facing each other.

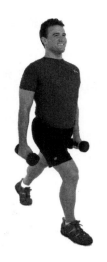

Raise your left leg by pushing it with your toes until your left thigh is parallel to the floor while simultaneously doing a biceps curl with both arms. This is one rep.

Reps: 8

Keep your arms as close in to your sides as possible. Your upper arms will barely move at all as you flex.

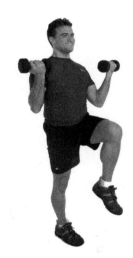

This Exercise Is Good for:

Brain: balance, coordination, multitasking limb movements, posture alignment, timing

Body: core strength; biceps, calves, front thighs, glutes, shoulders

5. Semi-Lunge with Upper Back Extension

Stand in the semi-lunge position, arms down comfortably between your hips and knees, palms facing each other.

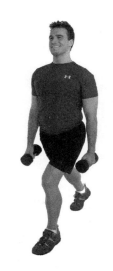

Raise your right leg by pushing it with your toes until your right thigh is parallel to the floor while simultaneously extending your arms straight up toward the ceiling. This is one rep.

Reps: 8

This Exercise Is Good for:

Brain: balance, coordination, multitasking limb movements, posture alignment, timing

Body: core strength; front thighs, glutes, shoulders, upper back

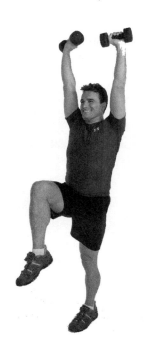

6. Semi-Lunge with Triceps Extension

Stand in the semi-lunge position, elbows bent at your waist, palms facing each other.

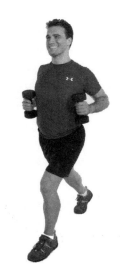

Raise your right leg by pushing it with your toes until your right thigh is parallel to the floor while simultaneously extending your arms back behind you. This is one rep.

Reps: 8

Keep your back straight at all times. You do not want to swing the weights or pull them too far back; the motion backward should be smooth and should feel comfortable.

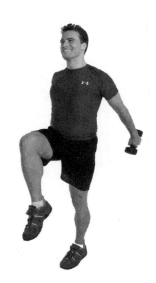

This Exercise Is Good for:

Brain: balance, coordination, multitasking limb movements, posture alignment, timing

Body: core strength; front thighs, glutes, shoulders, triceps, upper back

7. Semi-Squat Plié with Reverse Backhand

In the semi-squat-plié position, raise your heels slightly off the floor. Hold your arms slightly higher than hip height, elbows slightly bent, palms close to and facing each other.

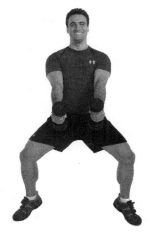

Extend your arms forward to slightly higher than hip height, palms close to and facing each other, and then move both hands to your left side, as if you were hitting a tennis backhand shot, slightly past hip level, without moving your head.

Repeat the movement, moving both arms to your right side. This is one rep.

Reps: 10

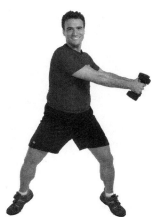

Your head should be straight at all times—not following the movement of your arms. If you feel it in your lower back, you're moving your head too much; you should feel the movement only on both sides of your waist.

Make sure you are perfectly balanced, with your heels raised, during the entire exercise. Do not raise your heels any higher than two inches off the floor or you might lose your balance.

Because most of the movement comes from your oblique abdominal muscles, you do not want to engage your hips at all.

This Exercise Is Good for:

Brain: controlled imbalance, coordination, multitasking movements (your lower body is balancing while your upper body is moving)

Body: core strength; back, front, and inner thighs; calves, chest, glutes, oblique abdominals, shoulders

8. Eyes Closed—One Leg Up + Biceps Curl

Stand straight with both feet close to each other, your arms straight at both sides.

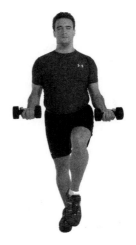

Close your eyes. Lift your left leg a few inches off the floor and raise your palms face-up to waist high, arms bent. Then, without losing your balance, raise the left leg until your left thigh is parallel to the floor while simultaneously doing a biceps curl. This is one rep.

Repeat on the other side, raising your right leg up off the floor followed by a biceps curl.

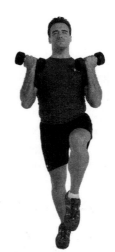

Reps: 5 with your leg stationary, followed by 5 with your leg moving up and down

Remember to keep your eyes closed. Open them only if you are losing your balance.

This Exercise Is Good for:

Brain: balance, coordination, posture alignment, sensory system

Body: core strength; back, back and front thighs, biceps, calves, chest, glutes, joints, shoulders

When your eyes are closed, your brain and body are missing their regular cues and must work much harder.

9. Opposite Arm and Leg Extension—Floor

Get down on your hands and knees on the floor, hands shoulder width apart, with your back straight.

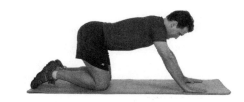

Simultaneously extend your left arm and your right leg.

Repeat on the other side. This is one rep.

Reps: 5

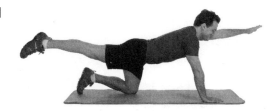

Do not raise your arm any higher than your shoulders.

Do not raise your leg any higher than your hips.

This Exercise Is Good for:

Brain: balance, coordination, multitasking limb movements, posture alignment

Body: core strength; back and front thighs, glutes, shoulders, upper back

10a. Crossed Leg with Push-up—Floor

Get down on your hands and knees on the floor, and then extend your right leg back. Without moving your upper body, cross your extended right leg over your bent left leg, tap it on the floor, and return to the starting position, with both knees on the floor.

Repeat on the other side, crossing your left leg over your right leg. This is one rep.

Reps: 8

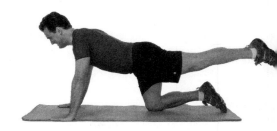

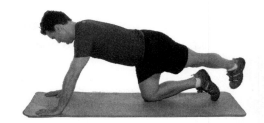

10b. Crossed Leg with Push-up—Floor

With your left leg still extended straight behind you, bend your upper body down into a half push-up.

Repeat the entire sequence on your right side. This is one rep.

Reps: 6

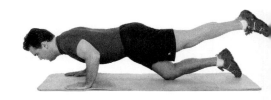

When you're doing the push-up, do not go down farther than a ninety-degree angle with your elbows. You don't need to do a full push-up.

This Exercise Is Good for:

Brain: balance, coordination, posture alignment, timing

Body: core strength; back thighs, chest, glutes, shoulders, triceps

11. Open Leg and Flies—Floor

Lie on your back with your legs up together and your feet pointing toward the ceiling, arms bent more than shoulder width apart, elbows almost touching the floor, palms facing each other.

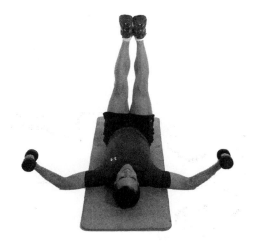

Raise your arms straight up, no more than shoulder width apart, while simultaneously opening your legs to form a V shape. This is one rep.

Reps: 8

Keep your arms slightly bent to avoid locking your joints.

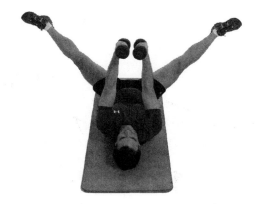

This Exercise Is Good for:

Brain: coordination, multitasking limb movements, timing

Body: abdominals, chest, front and inner thighs, glutes, shoulders, triceps

12. Bent Leg Sit-up with Flies

Lie on your back, with your knees bent up at a ninety-degree angle and your feet in the air, arms at ninety degrees from your torso and bent at a ninety-degree angle, elbows touching the floor, palms facing each other. Keep your head flat on the floor.

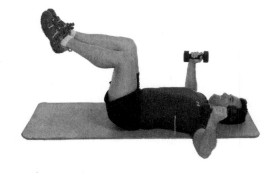

Lift your upper body off the floor while simultaneously raising your arms straight up, no more than shoulder width apart. This is one rep.

Reps: 8

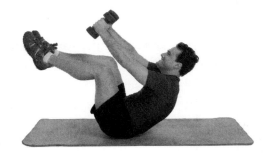

Do not look forward. Keep your eyes focused on the ceiling at all times.

If you feel a pull in your neck while doing the second step, you are not yet strong enough to raise yourself off the floor. Keep your head on the ground at all times until your core muscles become stronger.

This Exercise Is Good for:

Brain: coordination

Body: abdominals, chest, front and inner thighs, glutes, shoulders, triceps

13. Pelvic Raise with Flies

Lie on your back, arms bent at ninety degrees from your torso and feet flat on the floor, more than shoulder width apart, elbows almost touching the floor, palms facing each other. Keep your head flat on the floor.

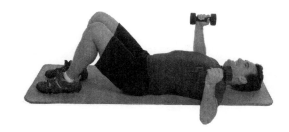

Lift your pelvis up as far as is comfortable while simultaneously raising your arms up, no more than shoulder width apart. This is one rep.

Reps: 8

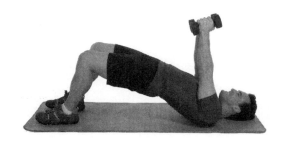

This Exercise Is Good for:

Brain: coordination, multitasking limb movements, timing

Body: abdominals, chest, front and inner thighs, glutes, shoulders, triceps

After you have done all the exercises, you will have finished one complete circuit.

Rest for zero to forty-five seconds, depending on your level, and then repeat the circuit two more times.

At the end of the third set, finish with a quick meditation cooldown. Ideally, you should aim for two to five minutes of meditation, but if you don't have time, even one minute will be extremely beneficial. Simply close your eyes, breathe deeply, congratulate yourself on the powerful work you have just done, and appreciate your strength and commitment. (Never judge yourself or be hard on yourself if you missed a movement or your circuit took longer than expected.) Then, mentally prepare yourself for the rest of your day.

8

Level 3: The Eagle

WOMEN

IF YOU ARE A BEGINNER

- Hand weights: 0–3 pounds
- Rest between circuits: 30–45 seconds
- Intensity: low-medium
- Approximate time per circuit: 3:30–4:30
- Approximate time per 3 circuits: 11:00–15:45

IF YOU ARE INTERMEDIATE

- Hand weights: 3–5 pounds
- Rest between circuits: 15–30 seconds
- Intensity: medium
- Approximate time per circuit: 3:00–3:30
- Approximate time per 3 circuits: 9:45–11:00

IF YOU ARE ADVANCED

- Hand weights: 5–7.5 pounds
- Rest between circuits: 5–15 seconds
- Intensity: medium-high
- Approximate time per circuit: 2:30–3:00
- Approximate time per 3 circuits: 7:45–9:45

If You Are an Athlete / Professional Player

- Hand weights: 7.5+ pounds
- Rest between circuits: none
- Intensity: high
- Approximate time per circuit: 2:00–2:30
- Approximate time per 3 circuits: 6:00–7:30

MEN

If You Are a Beginner

- Hand weights: 0–3 pounds
- Rest between circuits: 30–45 seconds
- Intensity: low-medium
- Approximate time per circuit: 3:30–4:30
- Approximate time per 3 circuits: 11:00–15:45

If You Are Intermediate

- Hand weights: 5–7.5 pounds
- Rest between circuits: 15–30 seconds
- Intensity: medium
- Approximate time per circuit: 3:00–3:30
- Approximate time per 3 circuits: 9:45–11:00

If You Are Advanced

- Hand weights: 7.5–10 pounds
- Rest between circuits: 5–15 seconds
- Intensity: medium-high
- Approximate time per circuit: 2:30–3:00
- Approximate time per 3 circuits: 7:45–9:45

If You Are an Athlete / Professional Player

- Hand weights: 10–12+ pounds
- Rest between circuits: none
- Intensity: high
- Approximate time per circuit: 2:00–2:30
- Approximate time per 3 circuits: 6:00–7:30

WOMEN and MEN

■ Follow the directions. Sometimes you'll start with your right leg and arm, sometimes with your left. All the circuits have been deliberately designed so that both sides of your body are worked out equally.

■ After two weeks of regular exercising, don't forget to gradually increase the amount of your hand weights. Never upgrade by more than 2 to 2.5 pounds. For example, if you start with 1-pound weights, your next weight can be 2 to 3 pounds; if you start with 3 pounds, your next weight will be 5 pounds.

■ If you have upgraded the amount of weights you're using and are ready to increase your level (from Level 6 to Level 7, say), drop the weight back down by at least 2 pounds. You can increase the amount of weights after two weeks of regular exercising. It's important to abide by this rule, because it will give you substantial muscular strength benefits without risk of injury.

■ It will take you a few days to master each circuit. Aim to reduce the time it takes you to do each circuit from the second week on.

■ For those who already have a regular cardiovascular routine, add these Super Body, Super Brain circuits after you've finished your cardio.

Level 3: THE EAGLE

STEP 1: MIND-SET

Visualize the exercises for thirty seconds before you start, just as a professional athlete would—with concentration, intensity, precision, and proper form. Say, "I am going to do my best. I know I can do it." Breathe deeply.

STEP 2: ALWAYS STRETCH BEFORE YOU START

Stretching not only loosens you up but sends a signal to your brain that you're ready to work out.

Standing tall and straight, place your feet slightly more than shoulder width apart. Raise both arms straight out at shoulder height, and then lean your body and your left arm to the left. You should feel the stretch in your waist.

Hold the stretch for fifteen seconds. Breathe deeply.

Return to center, and then repeat on the right side.

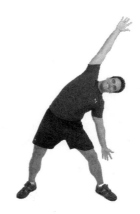

STEP 3: **ENERGY BOOSTER: CLAP + BALANCE**

You can do this exercise whenever you feel sluggish during the day, too.

From a semi-squat-plié position, with your arms down at your sides, clap between your legs.

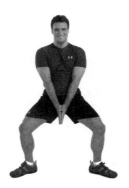

Stand up, and then raise your heels while simultaneously raising your arms to clap overhead. Don't forget to smile!

Reps: 10

Every count should be coordinated with a loud voice. You can count from one to ten or shout out positive ideas like "Let's do it," "We can do it," and "Come on."

Do your clapping with as much speed as possible.

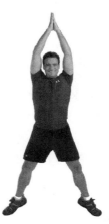

STEP 4: **EXERCISE CIRCUITS**

1. Opposite Leg Raise with Biceps Curl—Chair

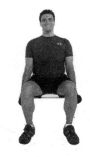

Sit tall on a firm, secure chair, chest out, core engaged by keeping your spine straight and your abdominal muscles pulled in, feet shoulder width apart, arms at your sides.

Stand up and do a biceps curl with your right arm while simultaneously bending your left knee up at a ninety-degree angle, foot parallel to the floor.

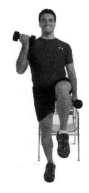

Sit down and return to the starting position.

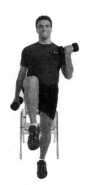

Repeat on the opposite side, doing a biceps curl with your left arm while bending your right knee up. This is one rep.

Reps: 5

The harder the surface, the better, so a chair is preferable to a sofa. If you do use a sofa, make sure it is as firm as possible.

Do not lean forward, since your posture needs to be impeccable at this level.

This Exercise Is Good for:

Brain: balance, coordination, opposite arm and leg movement, posture alignment

Body: core strength; front thighs, glutes, shoulders

2a. Leg Kick with Biceps Curl / Step Back and Forth

Stand tall, with your feet shoulder width apart, arms down at your sides. Cross your left leg slightly behind your right.

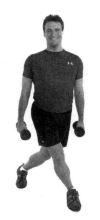

Kick your left leg out to the side while simultaneously doing biceps curls with both arms.

Change legs, and repeat on the other side. This is one rep.

Reps: 10

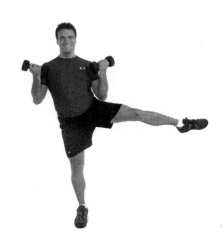

Ideally, these steps should be performed as quickly as possible, without losing the pattern. If you miss a step here and there, you're going too fast.

This Exercise Is Good for:

Brain: balance, coordination, footwork, speed, timing

Body: core strength; calves, front thighs, glutes, shoulders

2b. Leg Kick with Opposite Punch / Tapping

Standing with both feet shoulder width apart, raise one foot slightly, and then quickly follow it with the other foot.

Reps: 10

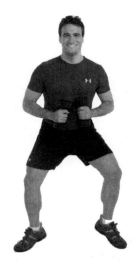

Think of the foot shift almost as a tapping movement, as if you were a basketball player defending your position.

Ideally, these steps should be performed as quickly as possible, without losing the pattern. If you miss a step here and there, you're going too fast.

This Exercise Is Good for:

Brain: balance, coordination, footwork, speed, timing

Body: core strength; calves, front thighs, glutes, shoulders

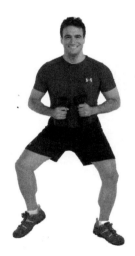

3. Seated-Standing Shoulder Raise

Sit tall on a firm, secure chair, chest out, core engaged by keeping your spine straight and your abdominal muscles pulled in, feet less than shoulder width apart, arms down by your sides, palms facing each other.

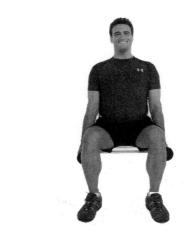

Stand up, and raise your left leg until your thigh is parallel to the floor while simultaneously extending your arms straight out to the sides.

Sit down again and repeat the exercise, raising your right leg. This is one rep.

Reps: 3

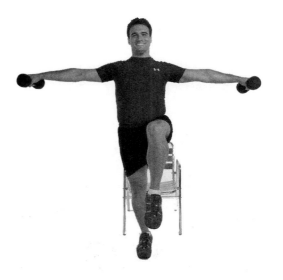

Be sure to keep your weight shifted back; you do not want to place your body forward over your knees. Your back should remain as straight as possible.

Do not raise your arms higher than your shoulders.

This Exercise Is Good for:

Brain: balance, coordination, multitasking limb movements, posture alignment, timing

Body: core strength; back, front, and inner thighs; calves, chest, glutes, shoulders

4. Seated-Standing with Biceps Curl

Sit tall on a firm, secure chair, chest out, core engaged by keeping your spine straight and your abdominal muscles pulled in, feet less than shoulder width apart, arms down by the sides of your thighs, palms facing forward.

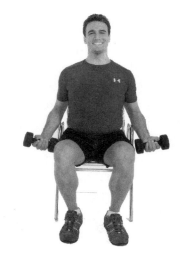

Stand up, and raise your left leg until your thigh is parallel to the floor while simultaneously doing a biceps curl using both arms.

Sit down again and repeat the exercise, raising your right leg while simultaneously doing a biceps curl using both arms. This is one rep.

Reps: 3

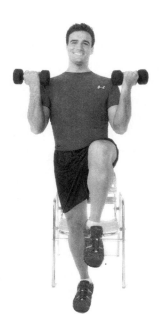

Keep your arms as close in to your sides as possible. Your upper arms will barely move as you flex.

This Exercise Is Good for:

Brain: balance, coordination, multitasking limb movements, posture alignment, timing

Body: core strength; biceps, front thighs, glutes, shoulders, upper back

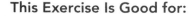

5. Seated-Standing with Upper Back Extension

Sit tall on a firm, secure chair, chest out, core engaged by keeping your spine straight and your abdominal muscles pulled in, feet less than shoulder width apart, arms down by your sides, palms facing each other.

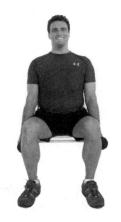

Stand up, and raise your left leg until your thigh is parallel to the floor while simultaneously straightening your arms overhead.

Sit down again and repeat the exercise, raising your right leg. This is one rep.

Reps: 3

This Exercise Is Good for:

Brain: balance, coordination, multitasking limb movements, posture alignment, timing

Body: core strength; front thighs, glutes, shoulders, upper back

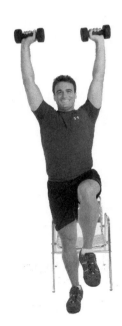

6. Seated-Standing with Triceps Extension

Sit tall on a firm, secure chair, chest out, core engaged by keeping your spine straight and your abdominal muscles pulled in, feet less than shoulder width apart, elbows bent so that both arms are at the sides of your waist, palms facing each other.

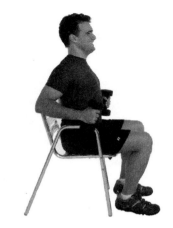

Stand up, and raise your left leg until your thigh is parallel to the floor while simultaneously extending your arms backward. Do not move your upper body forward.

Sit down again and repeat the exercise, raising your right leg. This is one rep.

Reps: 3

Keep your back straight at all times. You do not want to swing the weights or pull them too far back; the motion backward should be smooth and should feel comfortable.

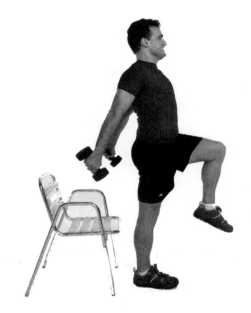

This Exercise Is Good for:

Brain: balance, coordination, multitasking limb movements, posture alignment, timing

Body: core strength; front thighs, glutes, shoulders, triceps, upper back

7. External Obliques—Flamingo

Stand tall, feet close to each other, holding one weight between both hands, and then raise your arms above your head, palms facing each other. Keep your arms straight above your head.

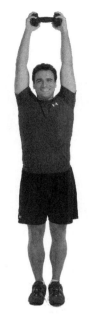

Raise your right leg to the side while simultaneously bending your waist to the right. This is one rep.

Reps: 5

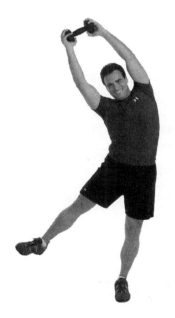

8. Eyes Closed—Biceps Curl + Upper Back Extension

Stand straight, both feet close to each other, your elbows bent at your waist, palms facing up. With your left foot slightly forward, raise your left leg.

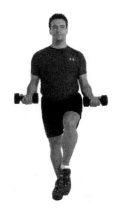

Bend your left knee, raising your leg as high as is comfortable. Do a biceps curl, and then straighten your arms above your head. This is one rep.

Change legs, then repeat.

Reps: 4

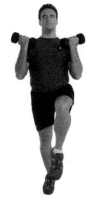

Try to keep your eyes closed. If this is too difficult, try closing only one eye at first.

Once you lift your foot off the floor, keep it off for the duration of the first and second steps.

When your eyes are closed, your body is missing its regular cues and has to work much harder.

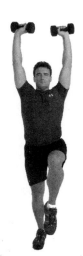

This Exercise Is Good for:

Brain: balance, coordination, posture alignment

Body: core strength; back and front thighs, biceps, calves, chest, glutes, middle back, shoulders

9. Eyes Closed—Opposite Arm and Leg Extension—Floor

Get down on your hands and knees, hands shoulder width apart, with your back straight. Close both eyes.

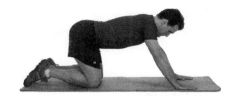

Simultaneously extend your left arm and your right leg.

Repeat on the other side. This is one rep.

Reps: 10

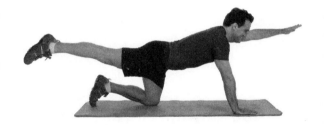

Do not raise your arm any higher than your shoulders.

Do not raise your leg any higher than your hips.

When your eyes are closed, your brain is missing its regular cues and has to work much harder.

This Exercise Is Good for:

Brain: balance, coordination, multitasking limb movements, posture alignment

Body: core strength; back and front thighs, glutes, shoulders, upper back

10a. Knee to Chest with Push-up—Floor

Get down on your hands and knees, and then extend your left leg horizontally behind you at hip height.

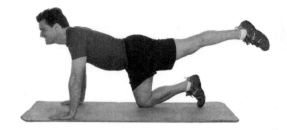

Bend your left knee and move your left leg up toward your head, rolling your back and lowering your head. This is one rep.

Reps: 8

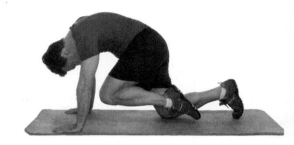

10b. Straight Leg Raise with Push-up—Floor

With your leg still extended up, bend your upper body down into a half push-up.

Repeat the entire sequence on your right side. This is one rep.

Reps: 6

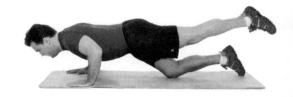

When you're doing the push-up, do not go down farther than a ninety-degree angle with your elbows. You don't need to do a full push-up.

This Exercise Is Good for:

Brain: balance, coordination, posture alignment, timing

Body: core strength; back thighs, chest, glutes, shoulders, triceps

11. Spread-Apart Legs and Triceps Extensions—Floor

Lie on your back, with your legs up and your feet pointing toward the ceiling, elbows bent at a ninety-degree angle, palms near your forehead and facing each other, shoulders and upper back raised no more than two inches off the floor, head flat on the floor.

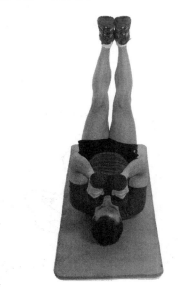

Spread your legs apart while simultaneously extending your arms straight out as if reaching for your legs. This is one rep.

Reps: 8

Be sure not to drop the weights on your forehead! If you can't hold them in the proper position without straining, use lower weights.

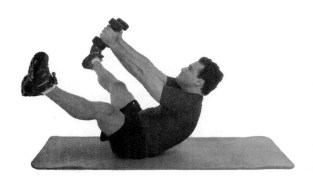

This Exercise Is Good for:

Brain: coordination, multitasking limb movements, timing

Body: abdominals, chest, front and inner thighs, glutes, shoulders, triceps

12. Bent Leg Sit-up with Chest Press

Lie on your back, your legs up and bent with your feet in the air, elbows bent at a ninety-degree angle, palms near your forehead and facing each other, shoulders and upper back raised no more than two inches off the floor, head flat on the floor.

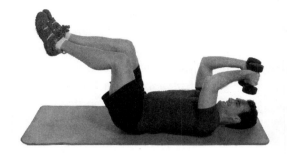

Lift your upper body off the floor while simultaneously raising your arms straight up and close to each other. This is one rep.

Reps: 8

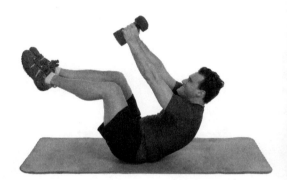

Do not look forward. Keep your eyes focused on the ceiling at all times.

If you feel a pull in your neck while doing the second step, you are not yet strong enough to raise yourself off the floor. Keep your head on the ground at all times until your core muscles become stronger.

This Exercise Is Good for:

Brain: coordination

Body: abdominals, chest, front and inner thighs, glutes, shoulders, triceps

13. Pelvic Raise with Chest Press

Lie on your back, with your knees bent at a ninety-degree angle, feet flat on the floor, elbows bent up at a ninety-degree angle. Place both palms, facing each other, on your forehead, and then raise them up two inches. Keep your head flat on the floor.

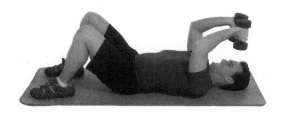

Lift your pelvis up as far as is comfortable while simultaneously straightening your arms upward, palms facing each other, no more than shoulder width apart. This is one rep.

Reps: 8

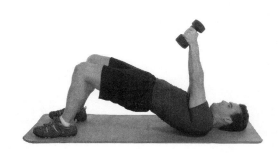

This Exercise Is Good for:

Brain: coordination, multitasking limb movements, timing

Body: abdominals, chest, front and inner thighs, glutes, shoulders, triceps

After you have done all the exercises, you will have finished one complete circuit.

Rest for zero to forty-five seconds, depending on your level, and then repeat the circuit two more times.

At the end of the third set, finish with a quick meditation cooldown. Ideally, you should aim for two to five minutes of meditation, but if you don't have time, even one minute will be extremely beneficial. Simply close your eyes, breathe deeply, congratulate yourself on the powerful work you have just done, and appreciate your strength and commitment. (Never judge yourself or be hard on yourself if you missed a movement or your circuit took longer than expected.) Then, mentally prepare yourself for the rest of your day.

9

Level 4: The Tiger

WOMEN

IF YOU ARE A BEGINNER

- Hand weights: 0–3 pounds
- Rest between circuits: 30–45 seconds
- Intensity: low-medium
- Approximate time per circuit: 3:30–4:30
- Approximate time per 3 circuits: 11:00–15:45

IF YOU ARE INTERMEDIATE

- Hand weights: 3–5 pounds
- Rest between circuits: 15–30 seconds
- Intensity: medium
- Approximate time per circuit: 3:00–3:30
- Approximate time per 3 circuits: 9:45–11:00

IF YOU ARE ADVANCED

- Hand weights: 5–7.5 pounds
- Rest between circuits: 5–15 seconds
- Intensity: medium-high
- Approximate time per circuit: 2:30–3:00
- Approximate time per 3 circuits: 7:45–9:45

IF YOU ARE AN ATHLETE / PROFESSIONAL PLAYER

- Hand weights: 7.5+ pounds
- Rest between circuits: none
- Intensity: high
- Approximate time per circuit: 2:00–2:30
- Approximate time per 3 circuits: 6:00–7:30

MEN

IF YOU ARE A BEGINNER

- Hand weights: 0–3 pounds
- Rest between circuits: 30–45 seconds
- Intensity: low-medium
- Approximate time per circuit: 3:30–4:30
- Approximate time per 3 circuits: 11:00–15:45

IF YOU ARE INTERMEDIATE

- Hand weights: 5–7.5 pounds
- Rest between circuits: 15–30 seconds
- Intensity: medium
- Approximate time per circuit: 3:00–3:30
- Approximate time per 3 circuits: 9:45–11:00

IF YOU ARE ADVANCED

- Hand weights: 7.5–10 pounds
- Rest between circuits: 5–15 seconds
- Intensity: medium-high
- Approximate time per circuit: 2:30–3:00
- Approximate time per 3 circuits: 7:45–9:45

IF YOU ARE AN ATHLETE / PROFESSIONAL PLAYER

- Hand weights: 10–12+ pounds
- Rest between circuits: none
- Intensity: high
- Approximate time per circuit: 2:00–2:30
- Approximate time per 3 circuits: 6:00–7:30

WOMEN and MEN

■ Follow the directions. Sometimes you'll start with your right leg and arm, sometimes with your left. All the circuits have been deliberately designed so that both sides of your body are worked out equally.

■ After two weeks of regular exercising, don't forget to gradually increase the amount of your hand weights. Never upgrade by more than 2 to 2.5 pounds. For example, if you start with 1-pound weights, your next weight can be 2 to 3 pounds; if you start with 3 pounds, your next weight will be 5 pounds.

■ It will take you a few days to master each circuit. Aim to reduce the time it takes you to do each circuit from the second week on.

■ For those who already have a regular cardiovascular routine, add these Super Body, Super Brain circuits after you've finished your cardio.

Level 4: THE TIGER

STEP 1: MIND-SET

Visualize the exercises for thirty seconds before you start, just as a professional athlete would—with concentration, intensity, precision, and proper form. Say, "I am going to do my best. I know I can do it." Breathe deeply.

STEP 2: ALWAYS STRETCH BEFORE YOU START

Stretching not only loosens you up, but sends a signal to your brain that you're ready to work out.

Standing tall and straight, place your legs more than twice your shoulder width apart, hands resting on your hips.

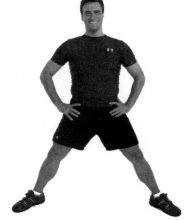

Bend your left knee, and then bring your torso down until you can place both hands on the floor near your left foot. You should feel the stretch in your extended right leg, which stays straight. Do not lock your knees.

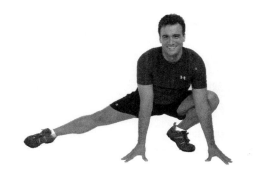

Hold the stretch for fifteen seconds. Breathe deeply.

Return to center and repeat on your right side.

STEP 3: **ENERGY BOOSTER: CLAP + BALANCE**

You can do this exercise whenever you feel sluggish during the day, too.

From a semi-squat-plié position, with your arms down at your sides, clap between your legs.

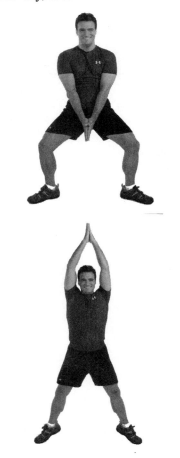

Stand up, and then raise your heels while simultaneously raising your arms to clap overhead. Don't forget to smile!

Reps: 10

Every count should be coordinated with a loud voice. You can count from one to ten or shout out positive ideas like "Let's do it," "We can do it," and "Come on."

Do your clapping with as much speed as possible.

STEP 4: EXERCISE CIRCUITS

1. Opposite Upper Back Extensions—Leg Straight to the Side

Stand tall, with you feet close together, arms at your sides.

With both elbows bent, straighten your left arm overhead while simultaneously moving your right leg straight out to the side.

Repeat with your right arm and left leg. This is one rep.

Reps: 15

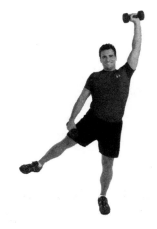

Keep the movement smooth, not jerky.

This Exercise Is Good for:

Brain: balance, coordination, opposite arm and leg movement, posture alignment

Body: core strength; front thighs, glutes, shoulders

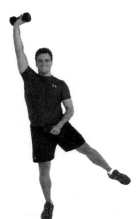

2a. Leg Kick to the Side with Biceps Curl + Leg Kick Front with Triceps Extension

Stand tall, with your feet shoulder width apart, arms at your sides. Cross your left leg slightly behind your right.

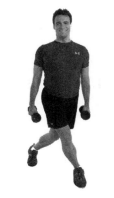

Kick your left leg out to the side while simultaneously doing a biceps curl. Then, without putting your foot down on the floor, do a front kick and a triceps extension.

Return to the starting position. This is one rep.

Reps: 8

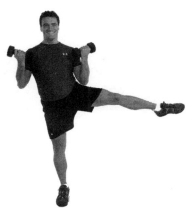

Keep your back straight at all times. Your posture needs to be impeccable and your movements smooth, since this is an extremely challenging movement.

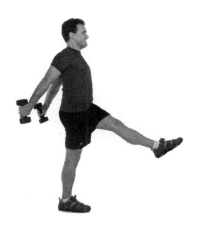

2b. Step Back and Forth + Tapping

Stand tall with your feet shoulder width apart, arms at your sides. Step about one foot forward with your left foot, and then bring your right foot up to it and parallel with it.

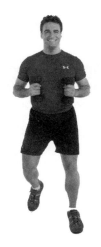

Move your left leg back to its original position and then follow with the right. These four steps are one rep.

Think of the foot shift almost as a tapping movement, as if you were a basketball player defending your position.

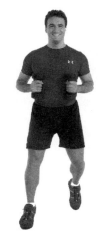

Ideally, these steps should be performed as quickly as possible, without losing the pattern. If you miss a step here and there, you're going too fast.

Change legs and repeat on the other side.

Reps: 10

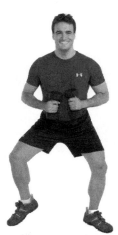

This Exercise Is Good for:

Brain: balance, coordination, footwork, speed, timing

Body: core strength; calves, front thighs, glutes, shoulders

3. Semi-Crossed Back Lunge with Shoulder Raise

Stand tall in the semi-lunge position, arms down comfortably between your hips and knees, palms facing each other. Cross your left leg behind your right.

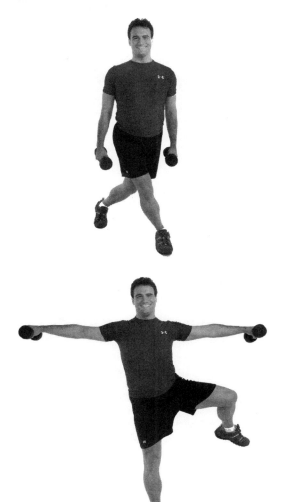

Raise your crossed leg behind you, and then bring it forward and to the side while simultaneously extending your arms straight out to the sides. This is one rep.

Reps: 8

Be sure to keep your weight shifted back; you do not want to place your body forward over your knees. Your back should remain as straight as possible and your hips facing front at all times.

Do not raise your arms higher than your shoulders.

This Exercise Is Good for:

Brain: balance, coordination, multitasking limb movements, posture alignment, timing

Body: core strength; back, front, and inner thighs; calves, chest, glutes, shoulders

4. Semi-Crossed Back Lunge with Biceps Curl

Stand tall in the semi-lunge position, arms down comfortably between your hips and knees, palms facing each other. Cross your left leg behind your right.

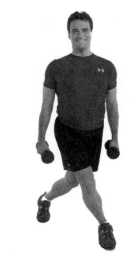

Raise your crossed leg behind you, and then bring it forward and to the side while simultaneously doing a biceps curl. This is one rep.

Reps: 8

Keep your arms as close in to your sides as possible. Your upper arms will barely move at all as you flex.

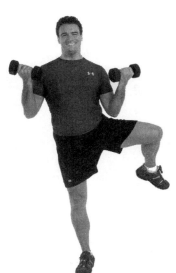

This Exercise Is Good for:

Brain: balance, coordination, multitasking limb movements, posture alignment, timing

Body: core strength; biceps, front thighs, glutes, shoulders, upper back

5. Semi-Crossed Back Lunge with Upper Back Extension

Stand tall in the semi-lunge position, arms down comfortably at your sides, palms facing each other. Cross your right leg behind your left.

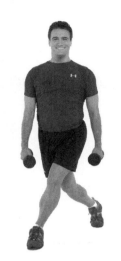

Raise your crossed leg behind you, and then bring it forward and to the side while simultaneously doing an upper back extension. This is one rep.

Reps: 8

Make sure your hips are facing front at all times.

This Exercise Is Good for:

Brain: balance, coordination, multitasking limb movements, posture alignment, timing

Body: core strength; front thighs, glutes, shoulders, upper back

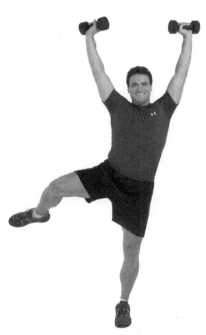

6. Semi-Crossed Back Lunge with Triceps Extension

Stand tall in the semi-lunge position, elbows bent, arms at both sides of your waist, palms facing each other. Cross your right leg behind your left.

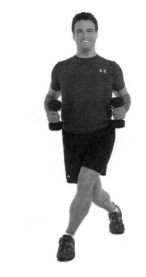

Raise your crossed leg behind you, and then bring it forward and to the side while simultaneously doing a triceps extension. This is one rep.

Reps: 8

Keep your back straight at all times. You do not want to swing the weights or pull them too far back; the motion backward should be smooth and should feel comfortable.

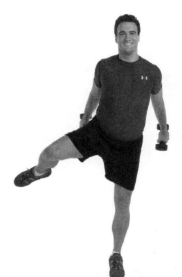

This Exercise Is Good for:

Brain: balance, coordination, multitasking limb movements, posture alignment, timing

Body: core strength; front thighs, glutes, shoulders, triceps, upper back

7. Semi-Squat Plié with External Obliques

In the semi-squat-plié position, raise your heels slightly off the floor, arms up and elbows bent at a ninety-degree angle at both sides of your head, palms facing forward.

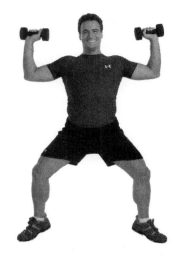

Extend your left arm overhead and to the right while simultaneously bending your waist to the right, without losing your balance. Keep your right arm in the starting position.

Repeat with the right arm. This is one rep.

Reps: 5

You should feel the pull in both sides of your waist.

Keep your heels off the floor during the entire exercise.

When your body weight shifts slightly to one side, you should move your head slightly to that side, too.

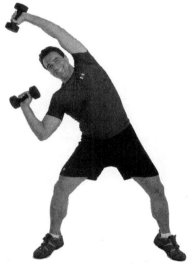

This Exercise Is Good for:

Brain: controlled imbalance, coordination, multitasking movements (lower body is balancing while the upper body is moving)

Body: core strength; back, front, and inner thighs; calves, chest, glutes, oblique abdominals, shoulders

8. Eyes Closed—One Leg Up—Biceps Curl / Leg Straight to the Side

Stand straight, with both feet close to each other. Close your eyes and breathe deeply, since this exercise will require maximum concentration.

Raise your left leg to the side while simultaneously doing a biceps curl. This is one rep.

Reps: 8

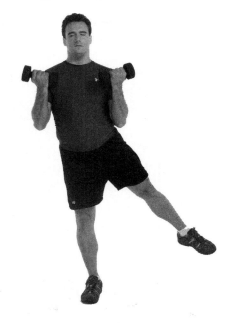

Do not let your foot drop to the floor.

Keep your back straight, since you must maintain impeccable posture alignment.

Make sure to keep your eyes closed during the entire exercise. Open them only if you feel you are losing your balance.

When your eyes are closed, your body is missing its regular cues and has to work much harder.

This Exercise Is Good for:

Brain: balance, coordination, posture alignment

Body: core strength; back and front thighs, biceps, calves, chest, glutes, middle back, shoulders

9a. External Obliques—Flamingo

Stand tall, feet close to each other, holding one weight between both hands, and then raise your arms above your head, palms facing each other. Keep your arms straight above your head.

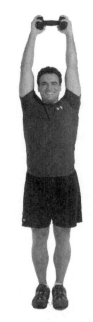

Raise your right leg to the side while simultaneously bending your waist to the right. This is one rep.

Reps: 5

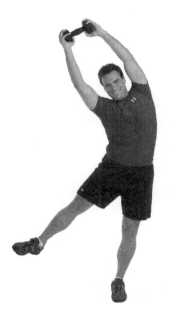

9b. External Obliques—Cross Behind Flamingo

Stand tall in the semi-lunge position, with one weight held in both hands above your head. Cross your right leg behind your left.

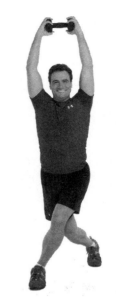

Raise your right leg to the side with your knee bent, while simultaneously bending your waist to the right. Return to the starting position. This is one rep.

Change legs and repeat entire sequence, starting with your left leg crossed behind your right.

Reps: 5

This Exercise Is Good for:

Brain: balance, coordination, posture alignment, timing

Body: core strength; glutes, internal and external obliques, quads, upper back

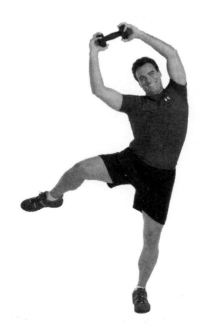

10. Opposite Arm and Leg Extension—Floor

Get down on your hands and knees, hands shoulder width apart, with your back straight. Close both eyes.

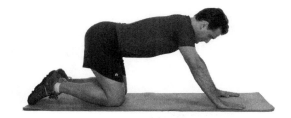

Simultaneously extend your left arm and your right leg.

Repeat on the other side. This is one rep.

Reps: 5

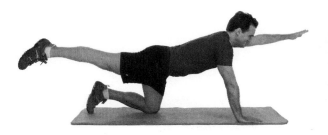

Do not raise your arm any higher than your shoulders.

Do not raise your leg any higher than your hips.

This movement should be as smooth and precise as possible.

Keep your eyes closed.

This Exercise Is Good for:

Brain: balance, coordination, multitasking limb movements, posture alignment

Body: core strength; back and front thighs, glutes, shoulders, and upper back

11. Legs Spread Apart and Chest Press—Floor

Lie on your back with your legs up and your feet pointed toward the ceiling, shoulders and upper arms slightly up off the floor, elbows bent up at a ninety-degree angle, palms facing forward.

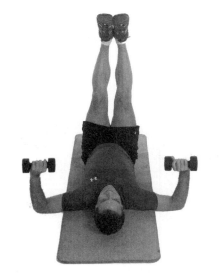

Open your legs while simultaneously bringing your upper body off the floor, and do a chest press while looking at the ceiling. This is one rep.

Reps: 12

Always keep your eyes focused on the ceiling.

This Exercise Is Good for:

Brain: coordination, multitasking limb movements, timing

Body: abdominals, chest, front and inner thighs, glutes, shoulders, triceps

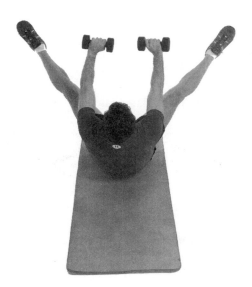

12. Face-Down Opposite Arm and Leg Raises

Lie face down, with your forehead on a soft surface, arms by your sides, toes on the floor.

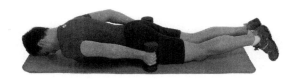

Raise your left leg two to four inches off the floor, as high as is comfortable, while simultaneously raising your right arm.

Return to the starting position, and then raise your right leg and left arm. This is one rep.

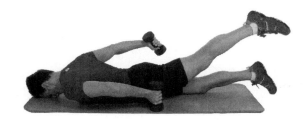

Reps: 10

This Exercise Is Good for:

Brain: coordination

Body: abdominals, chest, front and inner thighs, glutes, shoulders, triceps

After you have done all the exercises, you will have finished one complete circuit.

Rest for between zero and forty-five seconds, depending on your level, and then repeat the circuit two more times.

At the end of the third set, finish with a quick meditation cooldown. Ideally, you should aim for two to five minutes of meditation, but if you don't have time, even one minute will be extremely beneficial. Simply close your eyes, breathe deeply, congratulate yourself on the powerful work you have just done, and appreciate your strength and commitment. (Never judge yourself or be hard on yourself if you missed a movement or your circuit took longer than expected.) Then, mentally prepare yourself for the rest of your day.

Once you have successfully completed Level 4, you can move on to the Level 5+ circuits, which are covered in the next chapter.

10

Level 5+ Workouts

Congratulations! Now that you've mastered the first four levels, you're like a professional athlete who's moved on from the regular season to the playoffs. You've already seen an improvement in all the elements of these exercises: balance, coordination, execution, motion, precision, speed, and strength.

The way to keep Super Body, Super Brain as fresh and potent as possible is simple. All you have to do is create your own circuits by combining different exercise levels.

Level 5+: SUPER BODY, SUPER BRAIN INTEGRATION ROUTINE

By now you have internalized and can easily perform the sequence of different exercises. A mere glance at the instructions and you will know what to do. A few tips:

■ Do the three circuits at least once every day, although at this level you will likely be doing at least thirty minutes of Super Body, Super Brain, either all at once or broken up as suits your schedule.

■ The time it takes you to do each circuit should not change from earlier levels. Work on perfecting your form.

■ Your maximum recommended hand-weight upgrade will be from a minimum of 2 to a maximum of 4 pounds, for both women and men.

■ Refer to the Master Circuit, which starts on the next page.

Level 5	Circuit 1	Circuit 2	Circuit 3
Week 1	Level 1	Level 2	Level 1
Week 2	Level 1	Level 2	Level 2
Week 3	Level 2	Level 1	Level 2
Week 4	Master Circuit for all 3		
Level 6	Circuit 1	Circuit 2	Circuit 3
Week 1	Level 1	Level 2	Level 3
Week 2	Level 2	Level 1	Level 3
Week 3	Level 3	Level 2	Level 3
Week 4	Master Circuit for all 3		
Level 7	Circuit 1	Circuit 2	Circuit 3
Week 1	Level 1	Level 3	Level 4
Week 2	Level 3	Level 2	Level 4
Week 3	Level 4	Level 3	Level 4
Week 4	Master Circuit for all 3		
Level 8	Circuit 1	Circuit 2	Circuit 3
Week 1	Level 1	Level 2	Level 4
Week 2	Level 2	Level 3	Level 1
Week 3	Level 3	Level 4	Level 2
Week 4	Master Circuit for all 3		

MASTER CIRCUIT

Now that you've mastered all the advanced levels, you deserve a round of applause! By now you're in excellent shape, with increased strength, power, balance and coordination, flexibility, and brainpower.

There are several changes to this routine:

■ The circuits will take no more than four to five minutes.

■ This workout is at an advanced level, and you will be sweating hard. Don't forget to do your breathing, your meditation, and a cooldown afterward.

STEP 1: **MIND-SET**

Visualize the exercises for thirty seconds before you start, just as a professional athlete would—with concentration, intensity, precision, and proper form. Say, "I am going to do my best. I know I can do it." Breathe deeply.

STEP 2: **ALWAYS STRETCH BEFORE YOU START**

Stretching not only loosens you up, but sends a signal to your brain that you're ready to work out.

Standing tall and straight, place your legs more than twice your shoulder width apart, hands resting on your hips.

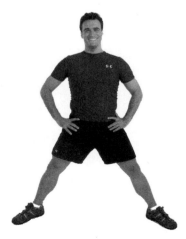

Bend your left knee, and then bring your torso down until you can place both hands on the floor near your left foot. You should feel the stretch in your extended right leg, which stays straight. Do not lock your knees.

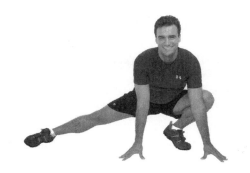

Hold the stretch for fifteen seconds. Breathe deeply.

Return to center and repeat on your right side.

STEP 3: **ENERGY BOOSTER: CLAP + BALANCE**

You can do this exercise whenever you feel sluggish during the day, too.

From a semi-squat position, with your arms down at your sides, clap between your legs.

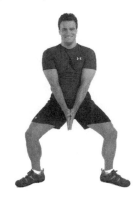

Stand up, and then raise your heels while simultaneously raising your arms to clap overhead. Don't forget to smile!

Reps: 10

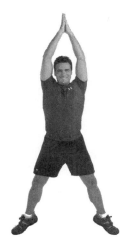

Every count should be coordinated with a loud voice. You can count from one to ten or shout out positive ideas like "Let's do it," "We can do it," and "Come on."

Do your clapping with as much speed as possible.

STEP 4: EXERCISE CIRCUITS

1. Opposite Arm and Leg Raise

Stand tall with your feet close together, arms at your sides.

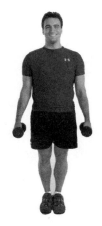

Raise your right arm above your head while simultaneously bending your left knee up at a ninety-degree angle, foot parallel to the floor.

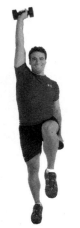

Repeat on the opposite side. This is one rep.

Reps: 12

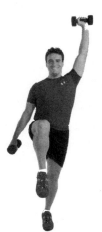

2a. Leg Kick to the Side with Biceps Curl + Leg Kick Front with Triceps Extension

Stand tall with your feet shoulder width apart, arms down at your sides. Cross your left leg slightly behind your right.

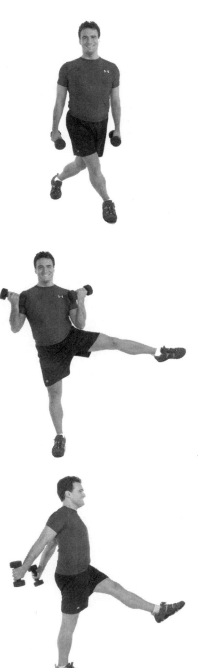

Kick your left leg out to the side while simultaneously doing a biceps curl. Then, without putting your foot down on the floor, do a front kick and a triceps extension. This is one rep.

Reps: 8

Keep your back straight at all times. Your posture needs to be impeccable and your movements smooth, since this is an extremely challenging movement.

2b. Step Back and Forth + Tapping

In the same starting position, step about a foot forward with your left foot, and then bring your right foot up to it and parallel with it.

Move your left leg back to its original position and then follow with the right. These four steps are one rep.

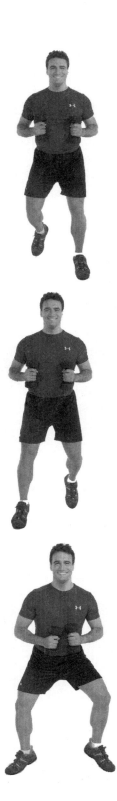

Change legs and repeat on the other side.

Reps: 10

Think of the foot shift almost as a tapping movement, as if you were a basketball player defending your position.

Ideally, these steps should be performed as quickly as possible, without losing the pattern. If you miss a step here and there, you're going too fast.

3. Semi-Squat Plié with Shoulder Raise

Stand tall in the semi-squat-plié position, arms down between your waist and knees, palms facing each other.

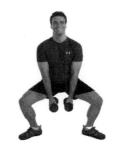

Raise your heels slightly off the floor while simultaneously extending your arms straight out to the sides. This is one rep.

Reps: 8

Be sure to keep your weight shifted back; you do not want to place your body forward over your knees. Your back should remain as straight as possible.

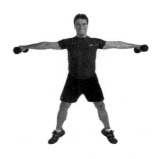

Do not raise your arms higher than your shoulders.

4. Semi-Lunge with Biceps Curl

Stand in the semi-lunge position, arms down between your waist and knees, palms facing each other.

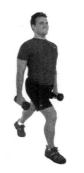

Raise your left leg by pushing it with your toes, keeping your heel slightly off the ground, until your left thigh is parallel to the floor while simultaneously doing a biceps curl. This is one rep.

Reps: 8

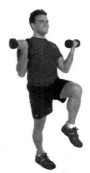

Keep your arms as close in to your sides as possible. Your upper arms will barely move as you flex.

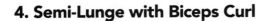

5. Semi-Crossed Back Lunge with Upper Back Extension

Stand tall in the semi-lunge position, arms down at your sides, palms facing each other. Cross your right leg behind your left.

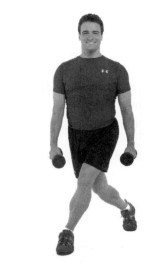

Raise your crossed leg behind you, and then bring it forward and to the side while simultaneously doing an upper back extension. This is one rep.

Reps: 8

Make sure your hips are facing front at all times.

For exercises 6, 7, and 8, repeat the sequences of exercises 3, 4, and 5, but change legs for exercises 4 and 5.

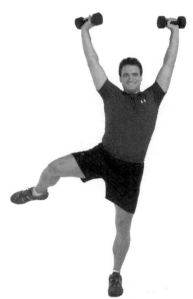

9. Semi-Squat Plié with Cross Jab

In the semi-squat-plié position, raise your heels slightly off the floor, arms raised to slightly below shoulder height, elbows bent at a ninety-degree angle.

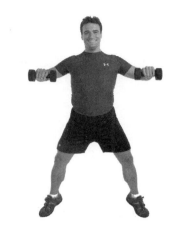

Extend your left arm across and forward to the right while twisting your waist to the left. Do not move your hips.

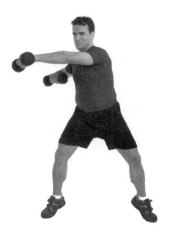

Repeat with the right arm. This is one rep.

Reps: 10

Make sure you are perfectly balanced, with your heels raised, during the entire exercise.

Do not raise your heels any higher than two inches off the floor or you might lose your balance.

Because most of the movement comes from your oblique abdominal muscles, you do not want to engage your hips at all.

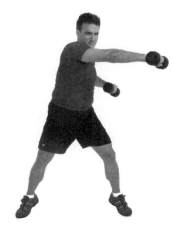

10. Semi-Squat Plié with Reverse Backhand

In the semi-squat-plié position, raise your heels slightly off the floor, arms raised to slightly higher than hip height, elbows slightly bent, palms close to and facing each other.

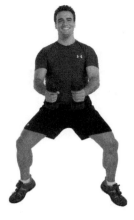

Extend your arms forward until the elbows are only slightly bent, and then move both arms to your left side as if you were hitting a tennis backhand shot, slightly past hip level, without moving your head.

Repeat the movement, moving both arms to your right side. This is one rep.

Reps: 10

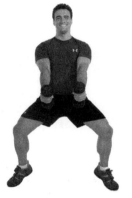

Your head should be straight at all times—not following the movement of your arms. If you feel it in your lower back, you're moving your head too much; you should feel the movement only on both sides of your waist.

Make sure you are perfectly balanced, with your heels raised, during the entire exercise.

Do not raise your heels any higher than two inches off the floor or you might lose your balance.

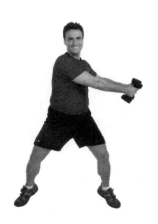

Because most of the movement comes from your oblique abdominal muscles, you do not want to engage your hips at all.

11. External Obliques—Cross Behind Flamingo

Stand tall in the semi-lunge position, with one weight held in both hands above your head. Cross your right leg behind your left.

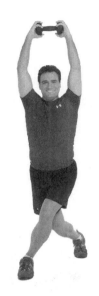

Raise your right leg to the side with your knee bent while simultaneously bending your waist to the right. This is one rep.

Change legs and repeat, starting with the left leg crossed behind your right.

Reps: 5

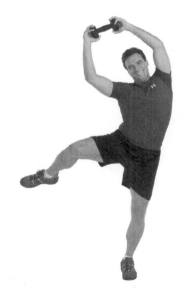

12. Eyes Closed—One Leg Up + Biceps Curl

Stand straight with both feet close to each other, arms bent at both sides of your waist, palms facing up. Bend your left knee, and then raise your left leg up off the floor as high as is comfortable.

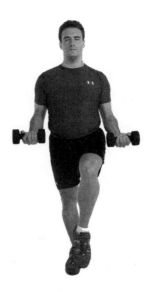

With eyes closed, do a biceps curl without losing your balance. This is one rep.

Repeat on the other side, raising your right leg up off the floor and following with a biceps curl.

Reps: 5 with your leg stationary, followed by 5 with your leg moving up and down

Remember to keep your eyes closed. Open them only if you are losing your balance.

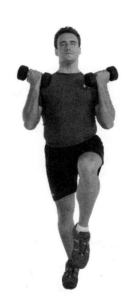

13. Eyes Closed—Biceps Curl + Upper Back Extension

Stand straight, with both feet close to each other, arms straight at both sides of your waist, palms facing up. Close your eyes. Bend your left knee, and then your left leg up off the floor as high as is comfortable.

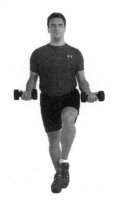

Alternate two arm movements: first, do one rep as a biceps curl; then, when your elbows are bent, straighten your arms above your head.

Return to the starting position. This is one rep.

Change legs, and then repeat.

Reps: 4

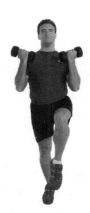

Try to keep your eyes closed. If this is too difficult, try closing only one eye at first.

Once you lift your foot off the floor, keep it off.

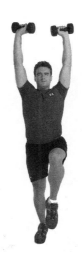

14a. Straight Leg Raise—Floor

Get down on your hands and knees, and then extend your left leg horizontally behind you to lower than hip height. Point your toes toward the floor so that your foot is at a ninety-degree angle to your leg.

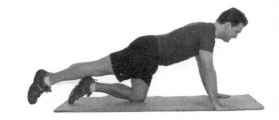

Raise your leg straight up no higher than hip height. This is one rep.

Reps: 8

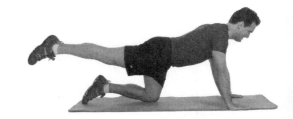

14b. Straight Leg Raise with Push-up—Floor

With your leg still up and extended, bend your upper body down into a half-push-up.

Repeat the entire sequence on your right side.

Reps: 6

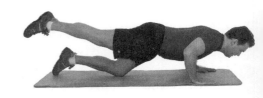

When you're doing the push-up, do not go down farther than a ninety-degree angle with your elbows. You don't need to do a full push-up.

15a. Crossed Leg—Floor

Get down on your hands and knees on the floor, and then extend your left leg back. Without moving your upper body, cross your extended right leg over your bent left leg, tap it on the floor, and return to the starting position, with both knees on the floor. This is one rep.

Reps: 8

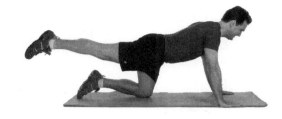

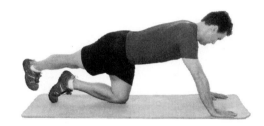

15b. Crossed Leg with Push-up—Floor

With your left leg still extended straight behind you, bend your upper body down into a half push-up.

Repeat the entire sequence on your right side.

Reps: 6

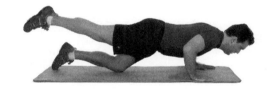

When you're doing the push-up, do not go down farther than a ninety-degree angle with your elbows. You don't need to do a full push-up.

16a. Knee to Chest—Floor

Get down on your hands and knees, and then extend your left leg behind you at hip height.

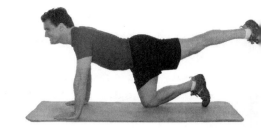

Bend your left knee, and then move your left leg up toward your head, rolling your back and lowering your head. This is one rep.

Reps: 8

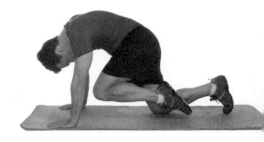

16b. Straight Leg Raise with Push-up—Floor

With your leg still extended up, bend your upper body down into a half-push-up.

Repeat the entire sequence on your right side.

Reps: 6

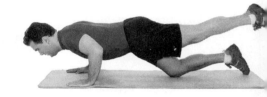

When you're doing the push-up, do not go down farther than a ninety-degree angle with your elbows. You don't need to do a full push-up.

17. Open Leg and Chest Press—Floor

Lie on your back with your legs up and your feet pointing toward the ceiling, shoulders and upper arms flat on the floor, elbows bent up at a ninety-degree angle, palms facing forward.

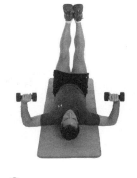

Open your legs while simultaneously extending your arms straight up no more than shoulder width apart. This is one rep.

Reps: 8

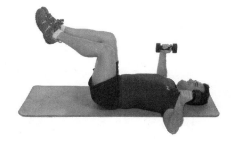

18. Bent Leg Sit-up with Flies

Lie on your back with your knees bent up at a ninety-degree angle, elbows bent up at a ninety-degree angle, shoulders and upper arms flat on the floor, palms facing each other. Keep your head flat on the floor.

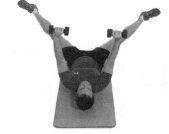

Lift your upper body off the floor while simultaneously raising your arms straight up, no more than shoulder width apart. This is one rep.

Reps: 8

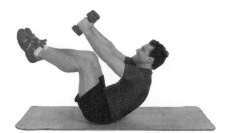

Do not look forward. Keep your eyes focused on the ceiling at all times.

If you feel a pull in your neck, you are not yet strong enough to raise yourself off the floor. If so, keep your head on the ground at all times until your core muscles become stronger.

19. Legs Spread Apart and Chest Press—Floor

Lie on your back with your legs spread apart to more than shoulder width, shoulders and upper arms flat on the floor, elbows bent up at a ninety-degree angle, palms facing upward. Straighten your arms upward at no more than shoulder width apart.

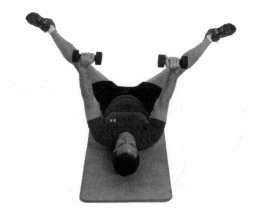

Bring your upper body off the floor and do a chest press while looking at the ceiling. This is one rep.

Reps: 12

Always keep your eyes focused on the ceiling.

After you have done all the exercises, you will have finished one complete circuit.

Rest for zero to forty-five seconds, and then try to repeat the circuit two more times.

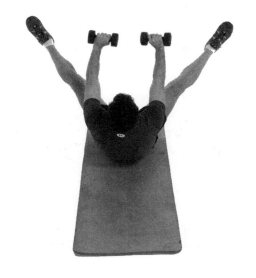

At the end of the third set, finish with a quick meditation cooldown. Ideally, you should aim for two to five minutes of meditation, but if you don't have time, even one minute will be extremely beneficial. Simply close your eyes, breathe deeply, congratulate yourself on the powerful work you have just done, and appreciate your strength and commitment. (Never judge yourself or be hard on yourself if you missed a movement or your circuit took longer than expected.) Then, mentally prepare yourself for the rest of your day.

Brain/Walking Circuit

Thirty Minutes to Boost
Your Brainpower

often joke with my clients who think they aren't coordinated that, in truth, they are. And the reason I know they are is very simple: they can walk.

Walking is one of the most amazing functions our bodies can perform—but it's also one that is invariably taken for granted. Sure, anyone can walk, but like any other physical activity, it takes only a very small amount of time and training to learn how to do it with even more skill. Once you master the basics of trained walking, you will be striding tall, with your head, neck, and back perfectly aligned; you'll engage more muscles, particularly those in your core; you'll strengthen your joints, ligaments, and tendons, particularly those in your knees, hips, and ankles; and you'll burn more calories.

The only equipment you'll need when you walk is a good pair of walking shoes that offer sufficient soft-tissue support. Therefore, I suggest that you find a good pair of shoes designed specifically for walking. If you're sore after your walks, especially around your ankles or heels, your shoes might not have enough support, and you should choose another pair.

Those of you who are advanced or experienced athletes and who have put in many miles walking can also consider carrying light weights to get an upper-body workout during your walks. And I mean light—no more than 3 to 5 pounds in each hand. But carry these weights only if they do not affect your postural alignment and you can stride as easily as you would if you weren't holding anything. You'll know the weights are too heavy if your lower back becomes sore or if you have discomfort in your ankles and/or knees. When you're holding the right weight, you won't have any soreness afterward.

Super Body, Super Brain Walk Training

Training yourself to walk is much more precise than merely cranking up your speed or swinging your arms more vigorously. One of the best exercises to improve your posture and alignment—one that you can easily do at home or outside on a hard, level surface (or even when waiting for a slow elevator to arrive!)—is to walk heel to toe. This brilliant little exercise literally trains you to walk perfectly. It works your hip stabilizers and strengthens the ligaments and tendons in your knees and ankles, which is helpful for anyone who has weakness in those joints. Even better, it's an exercise that every family member can do, and you need only a very small space with a level floor to do it in.

Thanks to our body's innate proprioception, you won't fall over when you do the heel-to-toe exercise. As you learned in chapter 1, your brain will be working hard to send the signals to the receptors in your muscles to keep your body upright, and your muscles will send the signals right back up to your brain.

I saw this concept in action when I was playing basketball in Spain and ankle injuries, particularly sprains, were extremely common. The trainers and physical therapists who worked with us always had us strengthen our sore ankles by having us get on a balance board with an unstable surface and then stand on one leg with our eyes closed. This was a terrific exercise in proprioception, since closing our eyes while striving to keep our balance robbed our brains of all visual cues, so our sensory system had to work that much harder to send and integrate all the signals from our proprioceptive receptors about where we were in space. Keeping this system functioning smoothly is what prevents you from falling over and injuring yourself.

I have practiced this exercise for over twenty-five hundred hours with many clients over the years, with a huge range in age and fitness level, and never had an ankle twist. Your body really is an amazing machine. Thanks to its innate proprioceptive skills, you will not fall over or twist your ankles while doing this exercise, even with your eyes closed. Should your body sense its balance to be out of whack, your eyes would automatically fly open and you would instantly right yourself.

Here's all you have to do to train yourself to walk:

■ **Place one foot** directly in front of the other, head up and eyes focused forward, in either an imaginary straight line or along the edge of a floor tile or board.

■ **Take six steps forward,** keeping your heels and toes aligned.

■ **Then do the same thing,** taking six steps backward.

Sounds ridiculously simple, right? But believe me, it's not as easy as it looks!

The key to doing this exercise properly is to fix your eyes on a point in the distance, precisely at eye level. You should not look down at your feet, which places undue stress on your neck muscles and throws your entire spine out of alignment.

But most people can't keep themselves from looking down. They not only fear taking steps without seeing what's in front of their feet, but don't understand the importance of correct postural alignment—which you can never have if your head and neck are turned down as you walk.

The reason that, when done properly, this is such a great alignment exercise is that you must engage all your muscles in order to stay on the imaginary straight line. This is the same principle as walking around with books on your head for balance. If you slump or look down, the books will fall.

It can take a bit of practice to walk this way, but you will soon see results and strengthen your core muscles as well as your joints in a safe, nonimpact way. You may need to keep your arms outstretched at first to keep your balance. Your goal is simply to walk in a straight line, head up, eyes forward, feeling strong and relaxed.

Try to do this for at least twelve steps, six forward and six back, at least three times.

Once you're better at it, try these heel-to-toe walking options:

- **Close your nondominant eye.** If you're right-handed, it's your left, and vice versa.
- **Close your dominant eye.**
- **Close both eyes** (as long as you're in a safe, enclosed space).

MORE ADVANCED:

- **Walk backward** without turning your head to see where you're going.
- **Add a hand weight** to each hand and do a biceps curl with each step.
- **Alternate arms** opposite to your legs (i.e., right leg, left arm).
- **Do the biceps curl** with arms opposite to your legs and with your eyes closed.

Boost Your Brain and Body by Walking

Walking improves your balance, coordination, gait speed, muscle efficiency, postural alignment, physical strength, and proprioception.

STEP 1: **MIND-SET**

Visualize the walk you're about to do for thirty seconds before you start: picture yourself having perfect postural and joint alignment, free-flowing energy, and physical strength. Say, "I am going to do my best. I know I can do it." Breathe deeply. Concentrating on your breathing will help with your postural alignment, too.

STEP 2: **ALWAYS STRETCH BEFORE YOU START**

Stretching not only loosens you up but also sends a signal to your brain that you're ready to start walking.

Stand tall, both legs wider than shoulder width apart, arms straight open at shoulder height.

Bend at the waist and drop your torso down so you can touch your knees, or farther if you can do so easily. If it's more comfortable, you can bend your knees slightly to avoid locking the joint.

You should feel the stretch in the back of your legs.

Hold this position for ten seconds, and then stand up straight and open your arms to the side while looking straight ahead. Then look up at the ceiling and breathe deeply.

STEP 3: **ENERGY BOOSTER: CLAP + BALANCE**

You can do this exercise whenever you feel sluggish during the day, too. And it's a great way to rev up your children.

From a semi-squat-plié position, with your arms down at your sides, clap between your legs.

Stand up, and then raise your heels while simultaneously raising your arms to clap overhead. Don't forget to smile!

Reps: 10

Every count should be coordinated with a loud voice. You can count from one to ten or shout out positive ideas like "Let's do it," "We can do it," and "Come on."

Do your clapping with as much speed as possible.

STEP 4: **WALKING CIRCUITS**

1. Warm-up

Walk at light intensity, with the same speed as if you were walking home. Swing your arms in a coordinated manner: every time you take a step with your left leg, swing your right arm, and vice versa. (The more pronounced your swing, the more your heart rate and coordination will increase.) Concentrate on your posture.

Stand tall, head erect, eyes focused forward. Do not look down.

Total time: 5 minutes

2. Interval Training 1

Circuit 1
Walk fast for 40 seconds, and then walk slower for 20 seconds.

When you walk fast, try to slightly increase your speed so you notice a significant difference between casual light walking and this speed. Faster walking will increase your heart rate and your muscle strength.

It's very important to breathe accordingly—meaning: the faster you walk, the faster and more shallow your breathing.

Reps: 5

Total time: 5 minutes

Circuit 2a
Do an opposite arm and leg raise for 30 seconds

Walk briskly for 30 seconds.

Reps: 3

Total time: 3 minutes

Circuit 2b
Walk while playing catch with a ball small enough to fit in your pocket. Throw the ball into the air, clap once, and catch the ball. Then throw the ball again and clap twice.

Alternate 2a's steps with 2b.

Repeat as many times as you can while maintaining proper postural alignment.

Total time: 3 minutes

Circuit 3
Walk fast for 30 seconds.

Stand tall, legs together, and then step to shoulder width with your left leg. Close up the step with your right leg and clap.

Reps: 10 starting with the left, then 10 starting with the right. Do this three times.

Total time: 4.5 minutes

3. Moderate Intensity Walk

Walk briskly, at moderate intensity. Concentrate on your posture. Stand tall, head erect, eyes focused forward. Do not look down.

Total time: 4.5 minutes

4. Interval Training 2

Circuit 1
With your arms completely extended in front of you, clap at head level while walking briskly.

Total time: 2 minutes

Circuit 2
Bring your arms up above your head and clap while walking.

Total time: 2 minutes

5. Cooldown and Stretching
Walk briskly for 5 minutes, gradually tapering down to the same light intensity you had during the warm-up. Your speed will decrease, and your breathing will become deeper and slower.

Stretch, as per the instructions in step 2 on page 182.

Standing tall, close your eyes and concentrate on your sense of accomplishment. Focus on your breathing, making a mental note of in and out. Do this for at least 2 minutes, since it is wonderfully calming.

Walking for Fitness

In addition to my thrice-daily Super Body, Super Brain sessions, I always make the time to do at least three cardio workouts every week. One of the best cardio exercises you can do is walking. It's low impact, it's easy to master, and it can be done practically anywhere—outside at the beach or in a park, or inside at a mall if the weather's bad. You can do it with friends, family, or even your dog (who needs the exercise too!).

Here's what happens in your body in a thirty-minute circuit.

Minutes 1–5

When you walk, you'll be using many different muscles in your legs, gluteus, core, arms, and shoulders.

Minute 6

Your stress hormones have increased in the bloodstream. These hormones are secreted from the adrenal gland, and their function is to help your cardiovascular system get blood, oxygen, and nutrients to your muscles and to make fat and glucose readily available to your muscles for energy production.

Minute 7

Low Intensity to Moderate Intensity: If you're walking slowly, your heart rate will barely have increased. It will still be beating at an average of 30 to 50 percent of your maximum heart rate. (See the heart rate formulas on page 55.)

Moderate Intensity: Walking with some speed will raise your heart rate up to 50 percent of its maximum, bringing more blood to your muscles. That means that your lungs will need to process more oxygen for use throughout your entire body.

Equally important, this heart rate is what's considered to be aerobic, which means your oxygen is constantly replenished in your working muscles.

A moderate heart rate is the ideal one, since you'll burn more calories while strengthening your heart muscle, without overtaxing your body. And one of the main benefits of training in the aerobic range is that it triggers the metabolism of your stored fat.

High Intensity: You'll be walking really fast, bringing your heart rate up to 75 percent of its maximum rate, which is when you'll leave the aerobic frontier and move into the anaerobic (no oxygen) territory. As a result, you'll be secreting more of the stress hormone cortisol and reducing your immune-cell functioning. This is not something I recommend during a fitness walk!

Minutes 8–9

If you're working out at moderate intensity, which for me is the best way to go, by minute 8 you'll see how efficient your entire motor system is. All your muscles will be perfectly coordinated, and your breathing will be strong and even.

If you are walking either too slowly or way too fast, it will be all too easy to forget your postural alignment, and you could tilt your neck forward, slacken your abdominal muscles as you arch your lower back, or pronate your ankles and/or knees (that is, turn or roll them inward).

Minutes 10–12

Ideally, you'll be walking somewhere that isn't perfectly flat. After all, not only is it more interesting to follow varied terrain, but going up and down hills works different muscles in your legs and core, too.

Having to walk up small inclines will slightly raise your heart rate and increase your blood circulation. At the same time, all your proprioceptors will keep on sending messages to your nervous system. If you're walking outside, you might see other people engaged in a variety of activities, traffic flowing (and crazy drivers driving), runners or cyclists moving, dog walkers walking, and more. In response, you're likely to vary your speed, which will also make your heart work well.

Minutes 13–14

You're nearly halfway there, and this is getting close to the dividing line between those who are aerobically fit and those who aren't quite used to this much exercise. Those who are beginners or who don't do regular strength training, such as the Super Body, Super Brain exercises, will start to feel tired. So even though they're determined to keep moving, they'll compensate for their fatigue by adjusting their posture and losing some of their good alignment.

Those who are stronger and more fit will feel energized at this point and should have

no difference in their posture or breathing rate.

Minutes 15–16

As with minute 13, walkers with powerful core strength will keep their pace and their form.

Minutes 17–19

At this part of the walk, when muscles start to experience fatigue, coordination becomes crucial. Inexperienced walkers will find it harder to maintain correct form; their upper body will move at a slower pace than their lower body.

Minutes 20–22

By minute 20, breathing patterns start to accelerate, even for experienced walkers. It's very important to focus on keeping your form as perfect as possible. It's better to slow down the pace a little while remaining posturally aligned than to rush and hunch forward.

Minutes 23–24

The rate and depth of your breathing continue to increase now. That's because as your muscles require more oxygen, the metabolic by-products produced by your working muscles need to be removed via your lungs.

Minutes 25–27

As your walking workout nears its end, you should gradually start reducing its intensity. But that doesn't mean you should slow down entirely. Ideally, you want to stay at a moderate intensity so you're still working your muscles aerobically. The more your body moves, the more oxygen will be required, and the more calories you'll burn.

Minutes 28–30

You should slow down for a few minutes, which will calm your heart rate and allow your breathing pattern to remain steady. You're likely to feel very good as your body releases neurotransmitters like endorphins and serotonin, producing a mental state of well-being.

Be sure to keep moving for a few minutes, until your heart and breathing rate are back to normal. You want to give your body a chance to slow down gradually. Don't forget to smile!

12

Super Body, Super Brain for the Family

When I was a child, I struggled with my weight. I was moody. I was clumsy. And I knew I would never be good at the sport I loved passionately if I didn't slim down. I was able to transform my own life—and I want to help you help your children transform theirs.

This is especially timely, because American children are facing a national health crisis. The number of overweight children has doubled, and the number of overweight adolescents has tripled, since 1980; 16 percent of children and adolescents age six through nineteen are overweight. As a result, type 2 diabetes has increased dramatically in youngsters, setting them up for a lifetime of complications and other health issues.

A study published in the *British Journal of Medicine* in 2008 showed that "children who showed poor hand control, poor coordination, and clumsiness at age 7 in testing were more likely to be obese adults. Those with poorer functioning motor skills at age 11 also tended to be obese at age 33."

There is also increasing scientific evidence showing a strong correlation between physical exercise and cognition, as discussed in chapter 1. Exercise can increase levels of brain-derived neurotrophic factor (BDNF) and other growth factors, stimulate neurogenesis, and contribute to brain plasticity in growing children, particularly through the late teens, when the cerebellum is still growing.

Child psychiatrist Gregory Lombardo, M.D., adds, "At younger ages, the brain has greater plasticity, so that the new learning is both easier, more exactly learned, and is more likely to have enduring effects on a child's future functioning."

But even as we know that getting enough physical exercise and movement is even more crucial for all children now, the terrible truth is that many children now live sedentary lives ruled by computers and video games and overburdened with academic demands, leading not only to poor health but to increased cases of stress, anxiety, and depression. According to the National Association of Sport and Physical Education, schools bowing to pressures from the federal government in terms of academic performance or that have lost funding often have no choice but to cut out gym class altogether. This is a scary concept, since lack of exercise and ensuing health issues are placing our children at risk for being one of the first generations to live shorter lives than their parents.

So I decided to do something about it.

The seeds of determination were planted when I'd go to my clients' homes in the late afternoon or evening, when the kids would be home from school and wanting their parents' attention. After one particularly gruesome afternoon of slammed doors and complaining, I had an epiphany: why not have the kids work out alongside their parents?

The results were instantaneous. Whining was replaced with wows. The kids were as challenged as their parents were, since they had to think while doing every single movement. Plus, they had the longed-for benefit of spending time having fun with their parents.

Super Body, Super Brain in Schools

Once I saw how well the children of my private clients were progressing, I realized that this program could easily be shared with larger groups of children—in schools. The more research I did about brain function and motor skills, under Dr. Lombardo's guidance, the more I realized I could develop a powerful program that could help children improve their motor skills, which would in turn improve their learning ability, memory retrieval, and academic achievement—and give them increased self-confidence.

The first school I worked in was PS 277, an elementary school in the Bronx, New York. The physical education teacher, Ms. Euridice Johnson, told me how difficult it was for her to get all students to participate in PE classes, since many of the students were too embarrassed by their lack of motor-skill dexterity to want to play sports.

I explained that all Super Body, Super Brain exercises were carefully designed with coordination challenges not only to improve motor skills but also to promote social interaction and very specifically to improve children's sensory systems and proprioception, two critical factors for brain development. Not only do children quickly master the movements, but the playful aspect makes them not seem like exercise. Without realizing it, when children are forced to think while doing any kind of movement, they're making their brains work harder, particularly linking the cerebellum (responsible for balance and coordination) to the frontal lobes (responsible for higher thinking and decision making). Their attention span increases while their fidgeting decreases.

Even more important for Ms. Johnson's concerns, the exercises are noncompetitive, so they work for all children, no matter what their size, shape, or innate athletic ability. Children who don't like sports or who've been teased for being uncoordinated will immediately be able to do the routines well, improving their self-confidence along with their motor skills. These exercises are the great equalizer.

What many coaches and school administrators don't realize is that school sports are often based on unique as well as advanced motor skills. At young ages, some kids have perfect mastery of these skills, but many kids don't—or they might be good at one kind of sport (like gymnastics or tennis) and not so good at another (basketball or soccer). Kids without advanced motor skills are usually branded as clumsy, uncoordinated, and useless for teamwork. Because these kids are usually teased and bullied and the last to be picked for teams, not only do they feel terrible about their athletic ability, but their sitting on the side-

lines gives them even less time to practice any skills. Being told that they're uncoordinated then becomes a self-fulfilling prophecy, setting these children up for a lifetime of inactivity and the belief that they're never going to be any good at exercising.

After a month of trying the program, Ms. Johnson called to tell me that all the kids were doing the same exercises, were sweating, and were having fun playing specific exercises that I designed to improve social interaction. Even better, a year later the Bronx district superintendent presented the results in an official report to the board of education, claiming that he saw "a remarkable improvement in the Physical Education Curriculum contributing not only to the children's physical condition and stamina but to their social interaction and a great impact in the classroom." The report added that the students improved 26 percent in reading and writing skills, showing a correlation between the exercises and their academic performance.

PS 277 principal Cheryl Tyler told me, "Your program gives students that possibility of succeeding—and this is why we like it."

Since 2008, I've trained over fifty PE teachers in New York, Pennsylvania, and Texas, and in Australia and Spain, in how to use my program, providing specific motor-skills-stimulating exercises for ages five and up. Because the school program starts out simple and develops more complexity only very gradually, no one feels left out—because no one is left behind. It's also wonderful that many children who found themselves on the bench soon develop enough motor skills to improve in a wide range of sports, too.

How Super Body, Super Brain Can Help Your Children

The Super Body, Super Brain exercises help children improve in the following different areas:

Motor Skills: Motor skills are movements that involve the use of the hands and precise hand-eye coordination. Since all the exercises actively engage motor skills, the balance and coordination that kids develop may help improve their brain functioning in attention, memory, multitasking, spatial memory, and decision making.

For example, repetitively raising heels and arms at the same time will improve attention and multitasking skills. This could correlate to better listening and/or handwriting skills in the classroom, or better multitasking skills, such as writing down dictation from the teacher.

Brain Stimulation: The cerebellum is the area of the brain responsible for voluntary physical movement, and it is connected by neurons to all parts of the cortex—the area

super body, super brain and neurological and learning disorders in children

One of the most potentially life-changing aspects of the brain is its capacity to rewire itself. This has profound implications for children who suffer from neurological disorders—from learning problems, attention disorders, anxiety, and depression to bipolar disorder or autism. Could their brains potentially be healed from within?

According to Dr. Lombardo, author of the book *Understanding the Mind of Your Bipolar Child*, bipolar disorder, which currently affects over four million children in America alone, is a condition afflicting the entire brain and, most important, the coordination of different parts of the brain. It's thought that fluctuating moodiness (as well as problems with reading and handwriting) are affected by poor integration of the brain's left and right hemispheres. The Super Body, Super Brain exercises advance gradually, so children imperceptibly learn to perform more and more complex exercises. As motor skills and balance improve, children's power of concentration and attention improve as well.

"This cannot help but improve problems with visual integration and with fine motor coordination and sensory-motor coordination," Dr. Lombardo explains, "yielding improvement is some children's reading and writing, both in the sense of handwriting and in the sense of composition."

Improved motor skills, balance, and coordination are particularly important for bipolar children, as well as those with ADD, as these children tend to be awkward, bullied, and isolated from group activities. They can do these exercises freed from any comparison with other children, since they're competing only with themselves. And because the exercises are fun, children don't see them as a chore, improving their skills without even realizing it.

of the brain responsible for higher-order thinking.

In addition, active children learn faster. In landmark studies that Charles Hillman and his colleagues published in 2009, they reported that physical fitness (specifically, aerobic capacity) improved cognition and brain function, often leading to improved academic achievement. Exercise appeared to prime the brain for optimal learning potential.

How well the information flows between right and left hemispheres is crucial for learning capabilities. Dr. Lombardo tells us: "We're finding that an increasing number of children have what's called a nonverbal learning disorder, which affects processing, and that, I think, in many cases has to do with poor or slow coordination between the right and left hemisphere. What Super Body, Super Brain is doing is deliberately increasing traffic across the hemispheres, and that traffic is cognitive as well as motor. I think this is something that can help some of the problems that kids have—not necessarily attention deficit disorder per se, but other learning issues that are mistaken for ADD."

Regular, movement-oriented exercise can also help some of the approximately fifteen million children with learning disabilities in this country. Dr. Eric Jensen, a pioneer scientist studying brain function and movement, concluded that movement, rhythms, physical activity, and exercise can help control many conditions such as ADHD, ADD, dyslexia, and hyperactivity—because movement helps facilitate a better integration between both brain hemispheres, improving balance, coordination, and concentration ability.

I am also working with several autistic children in New York City. Dr. Lombardo says, "The severity and the range of symptoms seen in children grouped under the diagnosis of autism can vary. However, one of the most common is difficulty with motor coordination and difficulty integrating movement with perception of space. Some clinicians believe that stereotyped movements, such as flapping, spinning, or head banging, are attempts on the part of autistic children to locate themselves in space or to manage the anxiety resulting from profound spatial disorientation. An important source of this disorientation is poor coordination of the left and right cerebral hemispheres, which affects three-dimensional vision, balance, motor coordination (both fine and gross), and the ability to maintain concentration while moving or while having to distinguish details in three-dimensional space."

The Super Body, Super Brain exercises improve integration of the right and left hemispheres, gradually building coordination, balance, and strength.

All children can benefit from exercise: it makes them feel better since it stimulates the release of endorphins, the neurotransmitters that make us feel good and that reduce the symptoms of depression. Exercise also tends to raise levels of the brain chemicals serotonin, epinephrine, and dopamine.

one family's super body, super brain experience

I met the Clausons when I was teaching workshops at the Mall of America in Minnesota in 2007, and I've stayed in touch with them over the years. It's been very rewarding watching their progress.

Brooke, age ten: "I like doing the workouts with my mom and sisters. The more I do them, the more energy I have. I think it has helped me to play better for my basketball team. I pay better attention when I am playing and get less tired running up and down the court."

Kayla, age thirteen: "My goal is to use the workouts to improve my posture and overall strength. I am not in any school sports, so it gives me a chance to be more active. I cross-country ski for fun, and the workouts have helped improve my balance and coordination. I might even join the school ski team next year."

Cassie, age sixteen: "Since I have started doing the workout, I've seen a lot of self-improvement. It has helped my endurance as well as my concentration levels. When I use it in the morning, it helps me pay more attention in school. It also has helped me improve my basketball game and lacrosse skills, and my coordination and my balance, too. The steps are fun and easy to follow, but it is an intense workout with great results."

Gary, dad, age forty-five: "Before I began doing the workouts, I was frequently tired during the workday. Since I have been doing the workouts my energy level has increased dramatically and I've been able to focus better at work. The exercises are engaging and make you think. Plus, I'm not as tired at the end of the day when I get home."

Amy, mom, age forty-three: "I never enjoyed going to a gym, as it was hard to fit into my schedule, nor have I been gifted with great balance or coordination—so Michael's exercises are perfect for me. They've helped me improve my core body strength and balance, and they're mentally engaging, unlike any of the other workout programs we tried and didn't like.

"We are a very busy family, and like most, it's a struggle to keep the kids off the TV and computer. But we now set limits and include the Super Body, Super Brain exercises in our household routine. It's awesome that this system combines three aspects—strength training, cardio, and mental stimulation—in the same program, and that our entire family can do it. My kids are so engaged with it that I no longer have to beg them to join in. Even better, I've seen improved motor skills, balance, and coordination in all of them. I also love that you do not need a lot of equipment for this program, so we can do it on vacations, too."

Cardiovascular Benefits: Cardiovascular benefits seen with any regular aerobic exercise are particularly important in school-age children.

Type 2 diabetes, caused by decreased physical activity and poor nutrition leading to obesity, has reached epidemic proportions in children. When children gain too much weight due to poor nutrition, particularly by eating a diet high in simple carbohydrates and fat and low in fruits and vegetables, the *number* of fat cells they have increases. (While experts once thought your number of fat cells was set at birth, they now know that it is possible to either lose existing fat cells or grow new ones. With adults, this number is fixed, but fat cell *size* is what increases.) Which means, unfortunately, that once children have an excessive number of fat cells, it becomes even harder to reverse obesity later in life.

Incorporating regular cardio exercise is important not only to burn calories and keep weight down, but for heart and circulatory health. I'd like to hope that the more a child exercises (and *likes* it), the more likely exercise will become a good habit for a lifetime.

You can easily add more fun physical activity into your entire family's daily routine, since the exercises here have been designed for parents to do together with their children. In only ten minutes a day, you will give your entire family incredible benefits for your brains and your bodies.

When Will My Kids See Results?

If you do only two or three sessions of no more than ten to twenty minutes each week, you will notice measurable results in as little as four weeks. But it's more likely that you will notice results right away as your children gain confidence, particularly as their motor skills improve, and a sense of pride in their accomplishment.

After ten weeks, you should expect to see:

- greater physical strength and endurance
- improved cardiovascular function and control of weight gain
- improvement in balance and coordination
- improvement in the perception of the body and its position in space
- improvement in concentration and attention
- improvement in self-esteem and mood
- reduced risk for sports injury
- lower blood pressure and resting heart rate
- more strength and stamina
- improved attention, concentration, learning skills, and memory
- increased ability to multitask

Parents/Children Super Body, Super Brain Circuit

Follow the directions. Sometimes you'll start with your right leg and arm, sometimes with your left. All the circuits have been deliberately designed so that both sides of your body are worked out equally.

■ Rest for twenty to thirty seconds between each exercise.

■ It may take you a few days to master this circuit. Don't worry; you'll soon be able to do all these exercises easily.

■ Make lots of noise! It's OK to sing, shout, holler, and whoop as you clap and move.

STEP 1: **MIND-SET**

Parents should help guide their children through this empowering visualization sequence.

Both of you close your eyes and visualize a beautiful park full of many fun things to do, and then visualize yourself lying down in the clean, green, sweet-smelling grass.

Concentrate on your breathing as follows:

For ten breaths, silently say, "In and out" every time you inhale or exhale.

Visualize your feet for ten seconds.

Visualize an orange for ten seconds.

Visualize a sun full of light, and end up with a smile that will transition to a loud laugh.

In every visualization, breathe deeply and say to yourself, "I am going to do my best. I know I can do it." Breathe deeply.

STEP 2: **ALWAYS STRETCH BEFORE YOU START**

Stretching not only loosens you up but also sends a signal to your brain that you're ready to work out.

Standing tall and straight, place your feet more than twice your shoulder width apart, arms at shoulder height and extended straight out.

Bend your torso down, and then reach down with your arms and touch your ankles.

Hold the stretch for ten seconds. Then, when you come up, say a loud "Ahh." Breathe deeply.

STEP 3: **ENERGY BOOSTER: CLAP + BALANCE**

You can do this exercise whenever you feel sluggish during the day, too.

From a semi-squat-plié position, with your arms down at your sides, clap between your legs.

Stand up, and then raise your heels while simultaneously raising your arms to clap overhead. Don't forget to smile!

Reps: 10

Every count should be coordinated with a loud voice. You can count from one to ten or shout out positive ideas like "Let's do it," "We can do it," and "Come on."

Do your clapping with as much speed as possible.

STEP 4: **EXERCISE CIRCUITS**

These exercises can all be done inside, in your backyard, or in a park.

All the Exercises Are Good for:

Brain: balance (proprioception and movement), concentration (multitasking), crossing the midline (left and right brain hemisphere integration), hand-eye coordination, kinesthetic awareness (knowing where your body is in space), sensory system / proprioception stimulation (particularly when eyes are closed)

Body: cardiovascular endurance; core strength; calves, front and inner thighs, glutes, hamstrings, postural alignment, shoulders

1. Monkey + Partners Clap

Pick a distance of ten feet between point A and point B. (Mark them with pillows if you like.) Face your child, standing three feet away.

In the semi-squat-plié position, clap your child's opposite hands ten times while jumping up.

Without stopping, move your body laterally as fast as possible to point B, and then clap your child's opposite hands ten more times. This is one rep.

Reps: 2

Kids under ten can make monkey noises while moving from point A to point B. (Parents and older kids can, too!)

2. Opposite Arm and Leg Raise

Stand tall, with your feet close together, arms at your sides.

Raise your right arm above your head while simultaneously bending your left knee up at a ninety-degree angle, foot parallel to the floor, and yell, "I am strong!" with each rep.

Return to the starting position, and then repeat on the opposite side. This is one rep.

Reps: 12

3. Hands on Shoulders, Knees Up

Stand tall, facing your child, and then place your hands on his or her shoulders.

At the same time, have both partners raise one knee up until it is bent at a ninety-degree angle, and then put it down and repeat with the other leg. This is one rep.

Reps: 10

Try to do this sequence as quickly as possible.

4. One Eye Closed—Leg Balance and Clap

Stand tall, facing each other, four feet apart. Both partners: shift your weight to your left leg, so that you're standing only on that leg. Close one eye.

Extend your right arm in front of you until you are able to reach your child's hand. Then clap each other's right and left hands. This is one rep.

Reps: 10, alternating hand claps with one eye closed

Repeat the entire sequence with the other eye closed. Then change legs.

Reps: 10

5. Stand Up and Down from Chair and Clap

Sit tall on a firm, secure chair, feet less than shoulder width apart, arms hanging loosely.

At "Go," stand up, raising your heels slightly off the ground while simultaneously clapping both hands overhead. This is one rep.

Reps: 5 with your eyes open and then 5 with your eyes closed

Sit back down and then stand up, bending your left knee up until your thigh is parallel to the floor while simultaneously clapping both hands overhead.

Reps: 5 with your eyes open and then 5 with your eyes closed

Hold each position for at least three seconds.

Alternate who says, "Go."

6. Pillow/Ball Throwing

Stand ten feet away from your child, and then throw a soft ball or pillow to the marker. This is one rep.

Reps: 10

Throw the ball or pillow with your heels raised slightly off the floor.

Reps: 10

Throw the ball or pillow with right knee bent up as high as is comfortable without losing your balance, and then alternate with your left knee bent and raised.

Reps: 5 with each leg

Repeat with one eye closed.

Reps: 5 with each leg

Throw the ball or pillow with precision, even with one eye closed.

7. External Obliques with Ball

Stand tall, back to back with your child, feet shoulder width apart and heels raised slightly off the floor, holding a soft ball or pillow, your arms extended straight in front of you.

Pass the ball or pillow from left to right.

Pass the ball or pillow to your child. Your child will pass the ball or pillow from left to right, passing the ball or pillow back to you.

Reps: 20

Keep your heels off the ground during the entire exercise.

Once you master this movement, do it as fast as possible without dropping the ball.

8. Snake: Stand Up at Go (Children Only)

Lie down on your back on the floor, arms and legs extended comfortably.

At "Go," jump up with as much explosive power as possible, clap opposite

hands with your parent, and then lie back down. This is one rep.

Reps: 10

Parents who are in good physical shape can do this with their children.

9. Extra Balance + Jump

Place a marker at least three feet away.

Stand tall, and then jump to the side with your feet together, like a frog, as close to the marker as possible, landing on both feet. This is one rep.

Reps: 10

Repeat, landing on one leg.

Reps: 8, alternating legs

10a. Balance and Count

Stand twenty feet away from your child.

At "Go," tell your child to go up on his or her tiptoes.

Slowly approach your child, flashing a number of fingers first with your left hand and then with your right. Your child should shout out how many fingers you're holding up while keeping on his or her tiptoes during the entire circuit.

Reps: 5

Once you can easily do this with both eyes open, repeat the exercise first with your left eye closed and then with your right.

10b. Balance and Read—Progression

After two weeks, add the following set:

Repeat exercise 10a, but change to word flash cards, alternating your left and right hands.

Reps: 5

Repeat step A, with one leg up as high as is comfortable.

Reps: 5

Repeat step A, with your left leg up and your right eye closed.

Reps: 5

Repeat step A, with your right leg up and your left eye closed.

Reps: 5

After you have done all the exercises, you will have finished one complete circuit.

Rest between circuits for up to a minute, and then repeat the circuit two more times, for three circuits total.

If you find the circuit to be easy, increase the number of circuits you do during each session, and reduce the amount of time between the circuits.

At the end of the third set, finish with a meditation:

Both of you close your eyes and visualize a beautiful park full of many fun things to do, and then visualize yourself lying down in the clean, green, sweet-smelling grass.

Concentrate on your breathing as follows:

For ten breaths, silently say, "In and out" every time you inhale or exhale.

Visualize your feet for ten seconds.

Visualize an orange for ten seconds.

Visualize a sun full of light, and end up with a smile that will transition to a loud laugh.

In every visualization, breathe deeply and say to yourself, "I am going to do my best. I know I can do it." Breathe deeply.

PART THREE

SUPER BODY, SUPER BRAIN

Eating Plan

13

Super Diet for a Healthier and Leaner Body

I t may be hard to believe now, but when I decided to stop playing basketball and immersed myself in my college classes, I went from buff to balloon. My weight zoomed up to an unbelievable 230 pounds, mainly because in my mind I was still an athlete working out six hours a day even though in reality I was a student immersed in my studies.

Worse, the cogent, focused mind-set that had fueled me forward for so many years disappeared. Instead of thinking about winning a basketball game, I had to switch gears entirely and focus on more sedentary academic pursuits—while managing a new kind of stress and anxiety. I "managed" by comforting myself with food.

Once I decided to whip myself back into shape, I did everything wrong. I did high-impact cardio for over an hour at a time and then lifted heavy weights, thinking that was the best way to burn calories. But the weight didn't come off—until I switched to the interval training my coaches had harped on about, combining short circuits done at medium intensity with lighter weights and high repetitions. *Bingo!* I never thought I could get ripped using only ten-pound weights. Even better, I saw impressive results after only three or four weeks, and had truly substantial gains after about four months.

But that weight loss wasn't due only to exercise. I had to change my attitude toward food. So I know how very difficult it can be to eat sensibly and nutritiously when faced with constant temptations. No matter how much exercise you do, if you don't watch what you eat—and if you eat more calories than your body truly needs—you'll still gain weight.

As you'll see, the weight-loss component of Super Body, Super Brain is as realistic as the exercises are. My goal is to have you target the kind of weight loss that will stay off, which means the weight-loss component needs to raise your metabolism through strength training (which builds lean muscle that burns more calories, even at rest) while lowering overall body fat.

I started working on a food plan when I saw my clients obsessively weighing themselves. I told them they'd feel a lot better if they stopped thinking about the word *diet*—which usually meant "deprivation" to them—and started thinking about foods that would be good for their bodies instead of the number on a scale.

At the same time that my clients were losing weight, they started eating more nutrient-dense foods targeted for their brains, too. Following the supercharged plan I developed with the marvelous nutritionist and registered dietician Olinka Podany, my clients were eating foods that would help them maintain a powerful brain, body, and bone structure.

What I also taught them, and what finally worked, was slow and steady weight loss—no yoyo diets, no deprivation, no crazy choices, no complicated menus and recipes, no expensive supplements. Just as the Super Body, Super Brain exercises progress gradually, making them easy to manage and giving you the language to build upon them, so should your weight-loss goals follow a gradual progression. It's much easier to cut 100 to 400 calories out of your diet over a period of weeks, for example—and adjust to that, and then slightly lower the calorie count again—than it is to make drastic changes that are impossible to maintain. And it is easier to make lasting changes if you begin to add targeted foods into your diet while making the choice to let go of some of your formerly favorite junk foods. By gradually implementing permanent changes into your lifestyle, you will develop a way of eating that will provide all the fuel you need to support both your body and your brain..

Let's start with the Super Body, Super Brain essentials.

The Right Amount of the Right Fats May Increase Your BDNF Levels

As you learned in chapter 1, BDNF, the neurotrophic growth factor in our brain, is something you want to have in abundant quantities for cognitive powers. One way to trigger BDNF production is through exercise. Another way is through food choices.

This means you need to rethink your attitude toward fat. Sure, you don't want a lot of fat in your diet since it's so calorie dense, but you do want to make your fat calories count to fuel both your brain and your muscles. Fats make up 60 percent of the brain and the nerves that run every system in your body. The membranes of your neurons are composed of fatty acid molecules. The protective sheath around your neurons is coated with myelin, which is 70 percent fat. Without adequate fat, your brain can't manufacture healthy brain cells. (Which is one of the main reasons that no-fat diets leave people feeling sluggish and cranky.)

The superfats your brain needs most are omega-3 fatty acids. Your body converts them into DHA (docosahexaenoic acid), which enhances brain communication. UCLA professor of neurosurgery and physiological science Fernandez Pinilla analyzed more than 160 studies on nutrition and your brain and became convinced that omega-3 fatty acids facilitate healthy plasticity between the synapses of your neurons.

Super "dud" fats are the omega-6 fatty acids (found in many oils such as corn and sunflower oil). Western diets contain too much of the omega-6 oils as well as way too much saturated fat, which clogs the arteries; omega-6 oils and saturated fat are linked to a higher risk of heart disease as well as Alzheimer's disease. Switching from nonnutritious saturated animal fats (like butter and lard) to healthier unsaturated fats (like olive oil) can also raise your BDNF levels. On the other hand, eating a diet with a chronically high level of saturated fat will destroy BDNF.

Smelling the Right Foods Can Trigger Neurogenesis in Your Olfactory Bulb

Every time you cook or eat, you should take the time to inhale deeply (unless of course you're about to eat some junk food!). This is because neuroscientists have proven that new nerve cells are created in the olfactory bulb, the area of the brain that governs your sense of smell, and we don't yet know everything about the wondrous new connections that might be formed.

Try testing your brain by smelling and tasting unfamiliar foods on a regular basis. The more flavorful the food, the more your olfactory bulb will be stimulated. But this means you should seek out flavorful, unprocessed, natural foods—like vegetables, fruits, herbs, and spices. Artificial aromas are nothing more than junk smells for your brain!

Knowing When Not to Eat

Your body is a machine the way your car is a machine: both need fuel. Your car needs gasoline, and your body needs calories. But when you park your car for the night, its need for gas is done for the day. Same with your body: it has little need for energy in the evening when you're getting ready to rest.

If you overeat right before bedtime, when you have little use for extra calories, you cannot possibly burn them all off as you sleep. Furthermore, if you consistently overeat at night, the accumulating calories not expended on energy can trigger an inflammatory response, because they are unused energy (calories not spent). And inflammation, as you know, can increase your risk of developing cardiovascular disease, diabetes, hypertension, and cancer.

My advice is to try to ingest most of your calories as early as possible during the day. Never skip breakfast (as you'll see in the section on page 214). Eat more at lunch than you do at dinner. And try not to eat more than an easily digestible snack (a piece of fruit, an unsweetened yogurt, for example) in the three hours before your regular bedtime.

How to Use This Chapter

This chapter is divided into two parts: Part 1 introduces the smart foods you want to eat that will not only maximize your brain's potential but provide the nutritional all-stars necessary for creating an incredible body. I will give you a smart food plan so you can have a super, lean, healthy body. Part 2 provides you with amazingly delicious, brain-smart, lean-muscle-building, low-fat and low-calorie recipes.

Part I: Super Brain Foods

Let's say you're about to approach a challenging mental task—giving a presentation, taking an exam, or interacting with your kids—and you're hungry beforehand.

Imagine eating a superfood (steel-cut oatmeal with blueberries), something that will nourish your brain and potentially give you an edge of mental sharpness, rather than some junk (sugary cereal) that won't. Follow through with that thought and imagine thirty minutes later and then an hour, after that meal choice. Can you see which is the better choice?

Many recent studies have shown that certain nutrients may have significantly positive effects on the brain. Ideally, a brain-healthy diet is one that encourages good blood flow to the brain, helps maintain mental sharpness, and reduces the risk of heart disease and diabetes. Adding smart food choices to your daily diet will help boost brain function, enhance memory, and improve concentration.

Smart steps to take:

■ **Increase your intake of protective foods.** Current research suggests that foods rich in antioxidants, which combat free radicals (substances that cause cellular damage), may reduce the risk of heart disease and stroke and appear to protect brain cells.

■ **Avoid multitasking while eating.** Enjoy your meal. Eat slowly and chew well. If you think of food not as the enemy lurking in wait to tempt you but as an important, nourishing element of each day, you will be better able to make smart choices about what to put in your mouth.

■ **Smell your food.** The olfactory bulb is one of the most important yet most puzzling areas of the brain, but as you learned in chapter 1, we do know that it is one of the areas capable of creating new neurons throughout adult life.

■ **Maintain a normal weight for the overall good health of your brain and body.** A long-term study of fifteen hundred adults found that those who were obese in middle age were twice as likely to develop dementia in later life. Those who also had high cholesterol and high blood pressure had six times the risk of dementia.

Smart Food Choices for a Better Brain

Here are some of the best food choices for brain function.

Apples

Two new studies from Cornell University suggest that apples may provide food for thought. Eating apples protects the brain from oxidative damage that causes neurodegenerative diseases such as Alzheimer's and Parkinson's. Quercetin is the phytonutrient in apples that appears to be largely responsible for the protective effect.

Asparagus, Spinach, and Leafy Green Vegetables

Your mother wasn't wrong when she told you to eat your vegetables, since leafy greens are particularly rich in folic acid, which is essential for the metabolism of long-chain fatty acids in your brain. Folic acid is also necessary for blood-cell formation. In addition, the antioxidants in spinach help reduce the risk of age-related decline in brain function. Researchers have found that including spinach in your diet may lessen brain damage from strokes and neurological disorders.

Beef

Beef is rich in vitamin B_{12}, iron, and zinc. Vitamin B_{12} helps maintain healthy nervous tissue and can also be found in eggs, fish, poultry, and dairy products. Iron is important because even a minor iron deficiency can impair concentration and mental performance; lean beef delivers one of the best absorbed sources of iron. Adequate zinc intake also plays a role in brain function. Even slight zinc deficiencies have been shown to impair memory.

Blueberries and Strawberries

Studies have shown that strawberry eaters may have a higher learning capacity and demonstrate better motor skill than non–strawberry eaters. Both blueberries and strawberries are full of antioxidants; a diet rich in such foods has been shown to boost the cognitive function of rats, and researchers at Tufts University speculate that similar results might occur in humans.

Dark Chocolate

Dark chocolate has powerful antioxidant properties. It also contains several natural stimulants, such as caffeine, that enhance concentration and stimulate the production of mood-enhancing endorphins. But don't see this as license to overindulge; the darker and less sweet the chocolate, the better, and half an ounce to an ounce a day is more than enough to provide benefits!

Eggs

Egg yolks contain choline. A choline deficiency may contribute to age-related mental decline and Alzheimer's disease. The nutrients in eggs support healthy brain tissue from birth to death. Choline becomes more important in preventing mental decline as we age.

Green Tea

Green tea contains a potent antioxidant, epigallocatechin gallate (EGCG), that appears to help fight cancer by stimulating apoptosis, a natural process in which the body destroys diseased or damaged cells but leaves the healthy cells intact. Green tea may also help protect against heart disease by lowering cholesterol and fighting coronary artery disease. In addition, several recent studies have found that EGCG has antiobesity effects, appearing to reduce body fat and waist circumference. EGCG is being studied for the prevention and treatment of Alzheimer's.

Olive Oil, Flaxseed Oil

As you read in the section about BDNF on page 202, your brain needs "good" fats. Olive oil and flaxseed oil are two of the best sources of omega-3 fatty acids, which enhance brain communication. (Just avoid heating flaxseed oil, since that destroys many of its nutritious properties.)

Prunes

Prunes are one of the most powerful of all antioxidant foods. They are also rich in fiber, potassium, iron, and vitamins B_6 and A.

Salmon, Other Oily Fish, and Flaxseed

Salmon contains the omega-3 fatty acids essential for all brain functions. Other oily fish are sardines, herring, trout, and yellowfin tuna. Flaxseed in the form of seeds or oil is an alternate source of omega-3s for vegetarians.

Spices: Dried Oregano, Ground Cinnamon, Ground Cloves, and Turmeric

Oregano, cinnamon, cloves, and turmeric are all potent sources of antioxidants. See the sidebar "About Antioxidants," on the facing page for more information.

Walnuts

Walnuts are rich in protein and contain omega-3 fatty acids, vitamin E, and vitamin B_6, making them an excellent source of nutrients for the nervous system. They are also high in potassium and other minerals such as zinc and iron. As with dark chocolate, moderate how much you eat. One tablespoon of walnuts is about five halves, with 50 calories and 5 grams of fat.

Whole Grains, Especially Oats and Barley

Whole grains deliver fiber and vitamin E, which helps promote good cardiovascular health. A healthy heart can provide good blood flow to the brain. The American Diabetes Association recommends oats because of the fiber content, and new research suggests that oatmeal may reduce type 2 diabetes. Barley is mineral rich, with particularly high levels of calcium and potassium, plus plenty of B-complex vitamins important for the nervous system. Research shows that both oats and barley have a cholesterol-lowering effect. The lower the cholesterol, the better your brain function.

Yogurt

Yogurt and other dairy foods are packed with protein and B vitamins essential for the growth of brain tissue, neurotransmitters, and enzymes. The active cultures in yogurt deliver additional benefits for bowel function. A healthy digestive system allows the brain to focus better and function effectively.

Anti-inflammatory Foods

As you learned in chapter 3, it's best for your health to keep inflammation in your blood vessels to a minimum, since this will allow for optimal blood flow to your brain, muscles, and all other tissues. Blood vessels clogged with cholesterol can cause heart disease and strokes.

But inflammation isn't a problem just for those worried about their cardiovascular health. Arthritis is a painful and debilitating disease that affects an estimated forty-six million Americans—that's nearly

about antioxidants

Antioxidants are critical for good health. They include a wide variety of plant-derived compounds; some vitamins such as C and E, some minerals, and flavonoids (compounds with antioxidant properties). The best sources of antioxidants are certain spices, fruits, and vegetables; flavonoids are also found in red wine and some teas. You can also buy antioxidants as supplements.

Antioxidants protect the body from damage caused by free radicals, which are substances in the body created as the by-product of cell functions and are implicated as a major contributing factor in the development of virtually all chronic and aging-related diseases. By neutralizing free radicals, antioxidants help prevent cancer, heart disease, and stroke.

Until more studies are done, you should get your antioxidants from a diet rich in fruits and vegetables, as well as from green tea or spices. No single antioxidant can provide adequate protection. The goal is to consume nine to eleven servings of fruits and vegetables each day.

one in five. It causes inflammation of the joints, which, in turn, can begin to limit your movement, leading to a cascade of ill health. So consider adding the foods on this list, all of which have anti-inflammatory properties, to help keep you moving.

Apples	Mung-bean
Artichokes	sprouts
Asparagus	Pineapple
Celery	Salmon
Cherries	Soybeans
Ginger	Spinach
Green tea	Turmeric
Leeks	Yogurt

You should also avoid the following foods if you're worried about inflammation:

• **Saturated fats,** since they contain chemicals called prostaglandins that cause inflammation, swelling, and joint destruction in rheumatoid arthritis

• **Excessive amounts of omega-6 fatty acids** (corn oil, sunflower oil, sesame oil, and wheat-germ oil), since they may promote autoimmune diseases such as rheumatoid arthritis

• **Nightshade vegetables** (potatoes, eggplant, peppers, and paprika), since they seem to be arthritis triggers

Prevention is key. If your cholesterol levels are elevated, take the American Heart Association recommendations seriously. Your total fat intake should be no more than 30 percent of your daily total calorie intake. Saturated fat should be 10 percent or less of your total calories.

Your Brain Needs Water, Too

Proper hydration plays a role in brain function because, as with inflammation, circulation is key. Your brain gets 20 percent of your body's blood flow every minute. So even if you're only mildly dehydrated, with perhaps a loss of no more than 1 to 2 percent of your body weight, this can affect how you feel and think, as all cells need a certain amount of hydration to function properly. Proper brain function requires eight glasses of water each day. (A glass is eight ounces.) This is often compounded by the fact that we develop an impaired thirst mechanism as we age, making it more difficult to gauge true thirst. Not surprisingly, those aged eighty-five to ninety-nine are six times more likely to be hospitalized for dehydration than those aged sixty-five to sixty-nine.

Dehydration does have an immediate effect on memory, producing confusion, difficulty thinking, and a general deterioration of mental performance. You'll feel tired, and your body temperature regulation will deteriorate, leaving you at increased risk for heat exhaustion and heat stroke.

If you aren't active, you still need to drink eight glasses of water each day. Those who engage in moderate to strenuous activity should consume eight ounces of water in the half-hour before exercise, three to four ounces every ten minutes or so during exercise, plus another eight ounces in the thirty minutes after exercise, whether thirsty or not.

Being well hydrated may also help you lose weight. Despite the fact that most diets tell you to drink those sixty-four ounces of water each day, few studies have been done to determine whether the practice actually speeds up weight loss. So researchers in Germany decided to do something about it. They found that after their subjects drank approximately seventeen ounces of water, the subjects' metabolic rates—the rate at which calories are burned—increased by 30 percent for both men and women. The increases happened within ten minutes of water consumption and reached a maximum after about thirty to forty minutes.

These researchers estimated that if you increase your water consumption by 1.5 liters (that's eight to ten glasses) a day over the course of a year, especially if it's cold water, you'd burn an extra 17,400 calories. This translates into a weight loss of approximately five pounds. The researchers found that much of the calorie burning was caused by the body's attempt to heat the ingested water. Though larger studies are needed to confirm this weight-loss effect, adequate hydration is clearly beneficial to your health. Drinking extra fluid even at room temperature is still beneficial for overall health.

Part II: Super Body Foods

Whenever I work in schools, I can't help but feel two contradictory impulses: I'm empowered and thrilled at seeing what children can accomplish in only a short time, quickly mastering the Super Body, Super Brain routines and clambering for more; and I'm depressed and frustrated that so many of these young children are already obese. I fear that they are doomed to a lifetime of eating issues because their parents have not yet taught them how to eat well. I know that the longer bad eating habits are entrenched, the harder it is to undo them. And the longer you live at an unhealthy weight, the harder it is to lose the excess pounds—and keep them off.

Obesity has been linked to most major diseases—unfortunately, often with results that have a terrible effect on your quality of life and can also lead to premature death. Excessive weight can cause heart disease, which can lead to congestive heart failure, sudden cardiac death, or a heart attack. It can cause diabetes; weighing just eleven to eighteen pounds over your ideal weight doubles your risk of type 2 diabetes. Extra pounds are associated with an increased risk of cancer of the colon, gallbladder, kidney, breast, and uterus lining. And each two-pound increase in body weight raises the risk of developing arthritis by 9 to 13 percent.

There's no magic bullet to get rid of excess weight. In fact, the formula, as you likely know already, is very simple: when you take in more calories than your body can metabolize through activity throughout the day, the excess calories are stored in your body. So you need to eat no more than your body can effectively use up, and you need to eat good, nutritious food while avoiding junk food, which gives you nothing but empty calories and health problems.

Usually, if weight suddenly starts to pile on, it's due to increased portion size and/or inactivity, although to rule out any underlying health conditions, you should always consult a physician if you are gaining or losing unusual amounts of weight.

Dieting can work as long as it's a realistic plan that won't trigger binges because you're hungry or bored by the same limited menu every day. Exercise also works, but not, of course, if you continue to overeat. Combining the two, however, yields a synergistic result: your weight loss will be faster, your health will improve more dramatically, and you will definitely look and feel a lot better. Weight loss is associated with a drop in blood cholesterol, meaning clean, healthy arteries better able to deliver nutrients and oxygen to the brain, helping it function better.

Keep in mind that weight loss is valuable *only* if it is permanent. We've all heard someone brag about losing a large amount of weight in a brief period of time; the problem is that the loss is usually followed by an even more astonishing weight gain once the strict diet regimen is tossed aside in favor of normal eating.

Your Daily Caloric Needs Formula

Use this formula to find your daily calorie level appropriate for weight loss:

target weight in pounds x activity level – age factor = daily calorie level

To find your activity level, multiply by 10 for light activity level, by 15 for moderate, and by 20 for heavy activity.

For the age factor, subtract 100 calories if you are thirty-five to forty-four; 200 calories if you are forty-five to fifty-four; 300 calories if you are fifty-five to sixty-four; and 400 calories if you are sixty-five or older.

For example, if you are thirty-six years old, if your target weight is 140 pounds, and if you are moderately active, your formula is $140 \times 15 - 200 =$ approximately 1,900 calories per day.

For most women, your daily calorie need will be between 1,200 and 2,000 calories, depending on how much weight you want to lose and how active you are. For men, the figure will be slightly higher.

Your caloric intake should never be *less* than 1,200 calories per day. Sure, you might lose a bit more weight in the short term, but in the long term you will send your body into starvation mode as it hoards the calories it is getting, slowing down your metabolism to conserve energy. As soon as you raise your calorie intake, your metabolism will still be more efficiently hoarding calories, and you'll quickly pile the pounds back on.

A healthy recommended weight loss is approximately one to two pounds per week. Not more! When you lose too much weight too quickly, you're not losing just fat, but muscle tissue, too. And that is exactly what you do *not* want to do, because muscle tissue is good. Muscle tissue is dense and healthy and weighs more than fat. It burns calories. In fact, one pound of muscle burns 35 calories each day, whereas one pound of fat burns only 2 calories each day!

And since one pound of fat is equal to approximately 3,500 calories, you can see how easy it is to gain weight. Add a few cookies that total 350 calories to your diet every day, and you'll gain a pound in ten days. And as we all know, it's much easier to pack on the pounds than it is to take them off.

Your goal is to maintain and/or increase your muscle mass—which will happen every time you do the Super Body, Super Brain exercises. Even if you choose to do only these exercises, and not diet at all, you will still lose some of your fat while building up your muscles. So even if your weight hasn't shifted a pound, your *shape* will have changed for the better.

It's easy to see how much you can transform your body through strength-training that builds muscle. Let's say you have ten new pounds of muscle instead of ten pounds of fat. You know that the muscle will burn 350 calories each day, whereas the fat would burn only 20 calories each day. As a result, your fit new body burns an extra 330 calories daily (350 − 20 = 330).

Most of all, don't compare yourself with anyone else. Your metabolism is unique to you.

Keep a Food Diary

Before you start any diet, it's a great idea to keep a food diary. Writing down what you eat each day practically guarantees weight-loss success. As with portion size, it's very difficult to know what, precisely, you're eating and drinking unless you pay careful attention—and most people are shocked to find out how much more they're eating than they need to. A food diary can be a tremendous help for those who've tried countless diets and failed: they really had no idea of the volume of calories they were inadvertently ingesting.

Not surprisingly, those who keep food diaries quickly become more self-aware about what they eat, when they eat, and why they eat. One study from the Kaiser Permanente Center for Health Research even showed that keeping a food diary was a better predictor of weight loss than exercise.

A good food diary should include when, what, how much, and why.

■ *When* tackles the timing of meals. Small, frequent meals are best. Many studies have shown that those who eat small, frequent meals eat fewer calories and fat grams than those who eat larger meals less often. This type of meal intake pattern keeps energy levels high and insulin levels steady. Small, frequent meals keep the blood glucose stable, preventing fluctuation and allowing the brain to function optimally without distraction.

Ideally, there should be six planned meals: breakfast, snack, lunch, snack, dinner, and snack, with a minimum of two hours between each meal. For example:

- 8:00 A.M.: breakfast
- 10:00 A.M.: snack
- noon: lunch
- 2:30 P.M.: snack
- 5:00 P.M.: dinner
- 7:00 P.M.: snack (no carb)

■ **What means you should record everything you consume:** all food, all drinks (even water), the mayonnaise on your sandwich, the hard candy you ate after dinner, even gum. Everything counts. An accurate record of your intake is essential.

■ **How much means portion size.** As you'll see in "Portion Size Matters," you should use measuring cups and visual cues until you've got the correct size pretty much as second nature. Size really does matter. Remember, double the portions equals double the calories.

■ **Why deals with your feelings about food.** Like portion size, they really do matter. Any kind of unusual eating behavior or cravings may be the result of circumstances and/or emotions that might need to be dealt with, and here you may be able to more readily see the brain–food connection. Write down everything you're feeling, and make note of your mental alertness throughout the day. This can be a tremendous help in identifying any triggers or associations you have with food. And remember, this is your private diary, and no one is going to see it but you (unless you want to share it with your physician).

I recommend that you keep a food diary for at least a month. Behaviorists believe that you need to stick to any new behavior for a minimum of three weeks while you get used to it and it can then become a permanent habit. After that, you can keep on making entries for as long as it's helpful.

Once you have this record of your eating habits, you can decide what you want to change. Start very small. Make gradual changes. As with the Super Body, Super Brain exercises, this is not a race. Your only goal is to have a strong and healthy body. As the old fable says, slow and steady wins the race—and weight loss and weight maintenance will be ongoing for your entire life.

Sit down with yourself and evaluate your successes or failures. Don't be hard on yourself if you didn't attain your goals. It can be very hard to manage your weight if you're under a lot of stress, traveling, or

Food Choices

You can mix your food choices as long as you stay within the same category.

	Monday	Tuesday	Wednesday	Thursday	Friday	Saturday	Sunday
8:00 am Breakfast							
10:00 am Snack							
noon Lunch							
2:30 pm Snack							
5:00 pm Dinner							
7:00 pm Snack							

SAMPLE SUPER BODY, SUPER BRAIN MENU

Meal Portion	Food
BREAKFAST	
1 fruit	1 cup berries
½ dairy	½ cup skim milk
1 starch	½ cup bran flakes
SNACK	
½ dairy	½ cup yogurt
1 fat	6 slivered almonds
LUNCH	
3 protein	3 oz. fillet of sole
2 starch	⅔ cup wild rice
2 vegetables	1 cup snap peas and onions
1 free food	fresh spinach and mushroom salad
1 fat	1 Tb. salad dressing
½ dairy	1 skim milk cappuccino

Meal Portion	Food
SNACK	
1 fruit	1 cup honeydew melon
½ dairy	½ cup plain yogurt
DINNER	
1 free food	1 cup clear broth
1 vegetable	4 oz. Virgin Mary
4 protein	4 oz. steak
1 starch	1 small baked potato
2 vegetables	1 cup broccoli
1 fat	1 Tb. gravy
SNACK	
1 dairy	1 cup plain yogurt

enjoying family celebrations. Just go back to basics and try again.

Portion Size Matters

Research has shown that Americans often underestimate how many calories they consume by about 25 percent. That's a lot of calories, and believe me, they add up—and the supersizing of portions is one of the reasons there's an obesity epidemic in this country.

I've actually seen people obsessed by every single calorie be brazen enough to haul out small food scales and weigh their food in restaurants. Although it's commendable to want to know what precisely you're eating when you go out, it's a lot more realistic to learn how much a serving size actually is and then to be able to eyeball it. The easiest way to do that is to use measuring cups and spoons at home, fill them with the proper-size portion of food, and then empty the food onto a plate. You will likely be shocked at how much food, particularly protein, you *don't* need!

You can also compare a portion size to a familiar object:

Pasta	Scoop of ice cream
Bagel	Hockey puck
Slice of bread	CD container
Steamed rice	Cupcake wrapper

breakfast brainpower

Many studies have found how important it is to eat breakfast, but I can't tell you how many of my smart, savvy, well-educated clients still skip that meal. That sets them up for binging as the day goes on, particularly at night. And it's even more important for children to eat breakfast—especially a nutritious one chock-full of whole grains, fiber, and protein (and low in added sugar) that can boost their attention span, concentration, and memory during a long school day. Research has also shown that children who eat breakfast ingest fiber, calcium, and other important nutrients. This meal more than any other helps them keep their weight under control, have lower blood cholesterol levels and fewer absences from school, and make fewer trips to the school nurse with stomach complaints related to hunger.

Try to eat a balanced breakfast that includes some carbohydrates, protein, and fiber. This will give you energy for your brain and muscles, and the fiber will make you feel full and stay full for longer. If you like cereal, read the label and aim for no more than 5 grams of sugar and at least 5 grams of fiber per serving. Drink lots of water, since the combination of water and fiber is what keeps your digestive system working smoothly to avoid constipation and bloating.

Don't forget how important it is to mirror good eating habits if you have children. Let your children see you taking time to enjoy breakfast every day. Even if you just wash down some whole-wheat toast and a banana with a small glass of juice or milk, you're showing them how important it is to face the day by refueling your brain and body with a healthy morning meal.

Meat, fish, poultry, tofu	Deck of cards
Raw fruit or vegetables	Baseball
Cooked fruit or vegetables	Your fist
Peach	Tennis ball
Cheese	Pair of dice

Don't forget to do portion sizing on anything you drink, too. Liquid calories count as much as solid ones, but they are equally underestimated if not forgotten completely!

Sugar Is Not So Sweet

You may have noticed that sugar isn't on my list of smart food choices—although it's often one of the most prevalent sources of calories, since the average American consumes about twenty teaspoons or more of sugar every day. That's very scary, since each teaspoon of sugar contains 16 calories, has no nutritional value whatsoever, and often causes cravings for more, even when you aren't hungry.

Do the math: a twenty-ounce bottle of soda has approximately 250 calories, all from sugar; that's the equivalent of sixteen teaspoons. You certainly couldn't eat sixteen teaspoons of sugar out of the sugar jar, could you? So if you do a bit more math, based on average sugar consumption, and calculate that $20 \times 16 = 320$ calories from sugar every day, you end up with an enormous 116,800 calories per year. That's nearly thirty-three and a half pounds!

Be aware of how insidious sugar is in most prepared foods, and realize that you've got to learn to read labels carefully, since sugar is often disguised in many forms. Look for the following: sugar, honey, corn syrup, high-fructose corn syrup, and words that end in *-ose* like sucrose, fructose, glucose, maltose, and lactose. Labels must list the amount of sugar in grams, and 4 grams of sugar is equivalent to one teaspoon.

Sugar abuse can lead to obesity, insulin resistance, out-of-kilter metabolism, and cavities. According to researchers, eating sugary foods can be bad for your blood vessels as well. A study published in the *Journal of Clinical Endocrinology and Metabolism* in August 2000 showed that when sugar is released into the bloodstream, free radicals, which can cause cellular damage, increased exponentially within two hours, while the level of natural vitamin E (a free radical–fighting antioxidant) dropped for three hours. This was a sign that the body was using vitamin E to deactivate the free radicals.

Although it is best to cut out table sugar entirely, that's highly unrealistic for most people. Sweets taste good. Restricting them completely means they become something to covet and obsess about. So I suggest you see sugar as a treat, to be eaten sparingly. It may be hard to believe, but once you cut your sugar intake, you really do lose your taste for it over time.

Low-Fat Eating

Eating too much fat can make you gain weight and feel sluggish, and if you're overweight there is no avoiding the fact that you will be more likely to develop heart disease, high blood pressure, diabetes, gallbladder disease, and many other health problems.

One of the big problems with fat is that it's calorie dense. One gram of fat contains 9 calories, whereas protein and carbohydrates contain only 4 calories per gram. Our tendency toward fatty foods is a remnant from the early years of our species, when food was scarce and our bodies needed to

nothing fishy

Fish is one of the most nutritious foods you can eat—as long as it's not fried! It delivers lean protein, B vitamins, and, if you pick the right type, heart-healthy and mind-boosting omega-3 fatty acids. The American Heart Association recommends at least two three-ounce servings per week, but watch out for fish high in potentially cancer-causing mercury.

THE WINNER: SALMON

Salmon is the highest in omega-3 fatty acids and the lowest in methyl mercury. It also provides B vitamins: B_{12} (a three-ounce serving exceeds the RDA), niacin, B_6, thiamine, and riboflavin.

FIRST RUNNER-UP: SARDINES

Just two little sardines give you a full day's worth of B_{12} and calcium. Sardines are also loaded with omega-3 fatty acids.

MORE RUNNERS-UP: COD, FLOUNDER, HADDOCK, SCALLOPS, SHRIMP, CRAB

All three of these white fish—cod, flounder, and haddock—are an excellent source of low-fat protein. A three-ounce fillet has only about 100 calories and one gram or less of fat. They are high in B vitamins and magnesium. All are low in methyl mercury. Flounder is your best bet for omega-3 fatty acids; cod and haddock contain less.

Low in calories and fat, shrimp have 85 calories per three-ounce serving, and scallops have 75; both have less than a gram of fat. Shrimp also provides 14 percent of your RDA of iron. Crab is an excellent low-fat, high-protein choice.

BOTTOM OF THE LIST: HALIBUT, TROUT, TUNA

Halibut, trout, and tuna are all rich in omega-3 fatty acids, iron, and magnesium but fairly high in methyl mercury. It is recommended that pregnant women and nursing mothers limit intake of fresh tuna and halibut to one serving a month, trout to six ounces a week.

OFF THE LIST: KING MACKEREL, SHARK, SWORDFISH, TILEFISH

King mackerel, shark, swordfish, and tilefish may be delicious, but they are all so high in methyl mercury that the FDA advises nursing women and those who are pregnant or are planning to become pregnant to avoid them. It is probably wise to skip this group and instead choose the smaller and therefore cleaner fish.

conserve as much fuel as possible. But we aren't hunter-gatherers anymore—unless you consider prowling through tempting grocery aisles a form of hunting!

Although the American Heart Association, the American Cancer Society, and the American Diabetes Association recommend that your daily fat intake be no more than 30 percent of your calories, most Americans get at least 50 percent of their calories from fat—and not from the "good" fats, either. In comparison, the typical fish- and carbohydrate-based Japanese diet gets approximately 10 percent of its calories from fat. The Japanese who eat this way have significantly less obesity, less heart disease, and less cancer, while those who have switched to a more Western-style diet are finding that their health and waistlines are suffering.

You can use this simple formula to figure out how many grams of fat you should eat each day, to try and keep your total intake under 30 percent of total calories: take your total daily calorie intake, calculate 30 percent of it, and divide that figure by 9 (the amount of calories per fat gram). This will be your daily fat gram number.

For example, assume that your daily intake is 1,800 calories; 30 percent of that is 540 calories. Dividing 540 by 9 gives you 60 grams of fat. Reading labels will give you an idea of the fat grams per serving of your favorite foods.

INSTANT FAT SAVINGS

INSTEAD OF:	Grams of Fat	TRY:	Grams of Fat
Doughnut	12	Raisin toast (1 slice)	0
Granola (1 cup)	15	Bran flakes (1 cup)	1
American cheese (2 slices)	16	Fat-free American cheese	0
French fries (large)	39	Baked potato	0
Fried rice (1 cup)	16	Steamed rice	0
Broccoli with cheese sauce	17	Steamed broccoli	0
Peanuts (½ cup)	56	Air-popped popcorn (1 cup)	0
Bologna (2 slices)	16	Turkey breast (2 slices)	1
Total grams of fat	**187**		**2**

One gram of fat = 9 calories; 187 grams x 9 = 1,683 calories from fat vs. 2 grams x 9 = 18 calories from fat. So you saved 1,665 calories in one day!

Super Body, Super Brain **RECIPES**

These recipes were developed by JoAnne Braganza, executive pastry chef of Recipe Consultants, Inc. (www.recipeconsultants.com), concentrating on super brain foods, anti-inflammatory foods, low-fat and low-calorie content, ease of use, and delicious taste!

Recipe Index

Breakfast

APPLE-CINNAMON OATMEAL

Serves 1

- **1 cup skim milk or water**
- **1 small apple, skin on, chopped**
- **½ teaspoon cinnamon**
- **¼ cup quick oats**
- **1 tablespoon chopped walnuts**

Add the skim milk, chopped apple, and cinnamon to a pot, and bring to a boil over medium heat.

When the skim milk reaches a boil, stir in the quick oats. Continue to cook for 1 minute, and then turn off the heat.

Stir in the walnuts.

YOGURT PARFAIT

Serves 1

- **1 cup fat-free plain yogurt**
- **¼ cup fresh blueberries**
- **2 medium strawberries, sliced**
- **2 tablespoons low-fat granola**

Place ½ cup of the yogurt in the bottom of a bowl or tall glass. Top with half of the blueberries and 1 sliced strawberry. Top with 1 tablespoon of granola. Repeat the layers of yogurt, berries, and granola.

GARDEN VEGETABLE FRITTATA

Serves 1

2 large eggs

1 teaspoon chopped Italian parsley

1/8 teaspoon kosher salt

1/8 teaspoon ground black pepper

1/2 cup washed, chopped russet potato, skin on

3 asparagus spears, chopped

2 tablespoons chopped red bell pepper, seeds removed

2 tablespoons chopped yellow onion

1 cup spinach

Whisk together the eggs, Italian parsley, salt, and pepper until well blended and foamy.

Preheat the oven to 400°F.

Heat a medium-size nonstick skillet over medium heat. Spray the bottom of the pan with canola pan spray.

Add the chopped potato and sauté for 6 minutes or until golden brown and tender. Stir occasionally to ensure even browning.

To the pan, add the chopped asparagus, red bell pepper, and yellow onion. Sauté until the vegetables are soft and tender, about 4 minutes.

Add the spinach and sauté for 1 minute, until the spinach just begins to wilt.

Pour the egg mixture evenly over the vegetables in the pan. *Do not* stir or the frittata may stick. Cook for 3 minutes or until the edges of the frittata begin to set.

Transfer the pan to the oven and bake for an additional 3 minutes or until the eggs are set and the frittata is puffed and golden.

WHOLE WHEAT BREAKFAST WRAP

Serves 1

2 large eggs
$\frac{1}{8}$ teaspoon kosher salt
$\frac{1}{8}$ teaspoon ground black pepper
1 cup spinach
$\frac{1}{4}$ cup chopped tomato
1 6-inch whole-wheat tortilla

Whisk together the eggs, salt, and pepper until well blended and foamy.

Heat a medium-size nonstick skillet over medium heat. Spray the bottom of the pan with canola pan spray.

Add the spinach and sauté for 1 minute, until the spinach just begins to wilt.

Add the chopped tomato and sauté for an additional minute.

Add the eggs to the pan. Using a rubber spatula, stir the ingredients occasionally to scramble the eggs.

Pour the scrambled egg mixture onto the center of the wrap and roll up.

Lunch

CHICKEN SALAD PITA

Serves 2

1 8-ounce boneless, skinless chicken breast

¼ cup chopped walnuts

1 medium apple, skin on, chopped

¼ cup chopped celery

2 tablespoons dried cherries

1 cup fat-free plain yogurt

¼ teaspoon kosher salt

¼ teaspoon ground black pepper

1 leaf romaine lettuce

1 4-inch whole wheat pita, sliced in half

Place the chicken breast in a pot and cover with cold water. Cook over medium heat, until the water comes to a boil. Adjust heat to medium low and poach the chicken for an additional 8 to 10 minutes or until completely cooked through.

Remove the chicken breast from the water and transfer to a plate. Place in the refrigerator and allow to cool for 10 minutes or until thoroughly chilled.

While the chicken is cooling, prepare the remaining ingredients. In a medium bowl add the chopped walnuts, apple, celery, dried cherries, yogurt, salt, and pepper.

When the chicken is chilled, chop and add to the bowl with the other ingredients. Mix to evenly incorporate all ingredients.

To assemble your pita, fold the romaine leaf in half and place into the pita pocket. Fill with half of the chicken salad.

Refrigerate the remaining chicken salad, and reserve it and the rest of the pita for a later time.

COLD POACHED SALMON SALAD WITH GINGER-SOY DRESSING

Serves 1

1 4-ounce wild salmon fillet, skin removed

¼ teaspoon kosher salt

¼ teaspoon ground black pepper

2 cups water

1 small lemon, cut in half

1 teaspoon finely grated ginger root

2 teaspoons olive oil

1 tablespoon reduced-sodium soy sauce

1 tablespoon orange juice

1 scallion, thinly sliced

2 cups mesclun lettuce

½ cup mung-bean sprouts

¼ cup shelled edamame

Season the salmon with salt and pepper on each side and reserve.

Place the water in a saucepan, and squeeze the juice of the lemon into the water. Bring to a boil over medium heat.

Once the water comes to a boil, reduce the heat to low and add the salmon. Simmer for 6 to 8 minutes, or until the salmon is completely cooked through. Remove from the water and transfer to a plate. Place in the refrigerator and allow to cool for 10 minutes or until thoroughly chilled.

While the salmon is cooling, prepare the dressing. In a bowl, whisk together the ginger root, olive oil, soy sauce, orange juice, and scallion.

To assemble, place the mesclun lettuce in a bowl and add the mung-bean sprouts, edamame, and chilled salmon. Top with the dressing.

BEEF AND BARLEY SOUP
WITH LEAN BEEF MEATBALLS

Serves 4

2 teaspoons olive oil

½ cup peeled, chopped carrot

½ cup thoroughly rinsed, chopped leek

½ cup chopped celery

1 cup button mushrooms, wiped clean and quartered

⅓ cup pearl barley

4 cups low-sodium beef broth or water

12 ounces 95 percent lean ground beef

2 cups spinach

½ teaspoon kosher salt

½ teaspoon ground black pepper

1 teaspoon dried oregano

In a medium-size pot, heat the olive oil over medium heat. Add the carrot, leek, and celery, and sauté for 6 minutes or until soft. Add the mushrooms and sauté for an additional 2 minutes. Add the barley and stir to incorporate.

Cover with beef broth or water and bring to a boil over medium heat. When the liquid reaches a boil, reduce heat and simmer covered for 35 minutes or until the barley is soft and tender.

Divide the ground beef into 12 small meatballs and add to the simmering soup. Cook for an additional 5 to 7 minutes or until the meatballs are cooked through.

Turn off the heat, add the spinach, and season with salt, pepper, and oregano. Serve immediately, or allow to cool and refrigerate.

WHOLE WHEAT PASTA SALAD

Serves 2

½ bunch asparagus, chopped
2 ounces whole wheat pasta, such as penne
8 ounces boneless, skinless chicken cutlets
⅛ teaspoon kosher salt
⅛ teaspoon ground black pepper
1 cup cherry tomatoes, cut in half
1 cup frozen artichoke hearts, defrosted
¼ cup Dijon mustard
1 tablespoon olive oil
¼ cup balsamic vinegar
6 leaves basil, chopped

Bring a large pot of water to a boil.

When the water is at a boil, add 1 teaspoon of kosher salt. Add the asparagus and cook for two minutes or until tender. Immediately remove to a bowl and cool under cold water. Drain well and reserve in a large bowl.

Return the water to a boil. Once the water is at a boil, add the whole wheat pasta and cook according to the manufacturer's instructions. Once the pasta is cooked, drain and cool under cold water. Drain well and add to the bowl with the asparagus.

Heat a grill or a sauté pan. Season the chicken cutlets with salt and pepper. Once the grill is hot, spray it with canola pan spray. Place the chicken on the grill and cook for 3 to 4 minutes on each side or until the chicken is cooked completely through. Remove from the grill and allow to slightly cool. Slice the grilled chicken into strips and add to the bowl with the asparagus and pasta.

To the bowl, add the cherry tomatoes and artichoke hearts.

In a separate bowl, whisk together the Dijon mustard, olive oil, balsamic vinegar, and basil. Pour over all the ingredients in the mixing bowl. Mix well to combine all ingredients. Serve at room temperature or chilled.

Snacks

ARTICHOKE AND SPINACH SPREAD

Makes 4 ½-cup servings

1 cup frozen artichoke hearts, defrosted
2 cups spinach
1 cup fat-free plain yogurt
½ teaspoon kosher salt
½ teaspoon ground black pepper
½ teaspoon cumin

In a food processor, add all ingredients and blend until well combined and the desired consistency is reached. Serve ½ cup of spread with whole wheat crackers or multigrain tortilla chips.

TURKEY, APPLE, CELERY, AND LOW-FAT CHEDDAR WRAPS

Makes 4 wraps or two servings

1 medium apple, skin on, cut into quarters
2 2-inch stalks celery, cut in half lengthwise
2 ounces low-fat cheddar cheese, cut into quarters
4 1-ounce slices deli-style lean turkey breast

Take one quarter of the apple and top with one quarter of the cheddar cheese and one slice of celery.

Wrap with one slice of turkey breast. Repeat with the remaining ingredients.

TRAIL MIX

Makes 6 ¼-cup servings

¼ cup low-fat granola
¼ cup dark-chocolate chips
¼ cup dried blueberries
¼ cup dried cherries
¼ cup walnuts
¼ cup almonds

In a medium plastic container with a lid, or in a food storage bag, combine all ingredients and shake to mix thoroughly.

GREEN TEA–BLUEBERRY SMOOTHIE

Serves 1

½ cup brewed green tea
½ cup blueberries
½ cup fat-free vanilla yogurt
2 tablespoons orange juice
½ cup ice

In a blender, combine all ingredients and blend until smooth.

Dinner

ROASTED WILD SALMON WITH COUSCOUS AND SPINACH–GRAPE TOMATO SALAD

Serves 2

1⅓ cups low-sodium chicken broth or water

¾ teaspoon kosher salt, divided

¾ teaspoon ground black pepper, divided

⅔ cup whole wheat couscous

2 6-ounce wild salmon fillets

2 cups spinach

1 cup grape tomatoes, cut in half

1 medium lemon, cut in half

Preheat the oven to 350 degrees Fahrenheit. In a small pot, bring the chicken broth, ¼ teaspoon of kosher salt, and ¼ teaspoon of ground black pepper to a boil.

Pour the couscous into a medium bowl. When the chicken broth has reached a boil, pour over the couscous and immediately cover with plastic wrap. Allow to sit covered for 10 minutes.

While the couscous is sitting, prepare the salmon. Season the salmon on both sides with ¼ teaspoon of kosher salt and ¼ teaspoon of ground black pepper. Spray a baking pan with canola pan spray. Place the salmon on the baking pan, and bake in the oven for 12 minutes or until the salmon is completely cooked through.

Uncover the couscous and fluff with a fork. Divide equally among two dishes.

In a mixing bowl, combine the spinach and grape tomatoes. Squeeze the lemon over the spinach and grape tomatoes, and add ¼ teaspoon of kosher salt and ¼ teaspoon of ground black pepper. Mix to combine.

Remove the salmon from the oven and place on top of the couscous. Divide the spinach and grape tomato salad evenly over the salmon.

MARINATED FILET MIGNON WITH GRILLED ASPARAGUS AND A CRUSHED YUKON GOLD POTATO

Serves 2

- 2 4-ounce filet mignon steaks, trimmed of outer fat
- 2 teaspoons chopped rosemary, divided
- 2 teaspoons chopped parsley, divided
- 1¼ teaspoons kosher salt, divided
- 1¼ teaspoons ground black pepper, divided
- 3 teaspoons olive oil, divided
- ½ bunch asparagus
- 1 medium lemon, cut in half
- 2 small Yukon gold potatoes

Bring a medium-size pot of water to a boil.

Place the filet mignon steaks in a medium-size bowl. Sprinkle with 1 teaspoon of rosemary, 1 teaspoon of parsley, ½ teaspoon of kosher salt, ½ teaspoon of ground black pepper, and 1 teaspoon of olive oil. Mix to coat the steaks well with all ingredients. Allow to marinate for at least fifteen minutes or up to 1 hour in the refrigerator.

Preheat your grill to 400 degrees Fahrenheit while the steaks are marinating. When the water reaches a boil, add the asparagus and cook for 2 minutes or until tender. Immediately remove to a bowl and cool under cold water. Drain well and sprinkle with ¼ teaspoon of kosher salt, ¼ teaspoon of ground black pepper, and the juice of the lemon. Reserve.

Return the water to a boil and add the Yukon gold potatoes. Cook for 15 minutes or until fork tender. Drain the potatoes well, and then crush them slightly with a fork until the skins crack and the potatoes flatten. Place both flattened potatoes on a sheet of aluminum foil, drizzle each with 1 teaspoon of olive oil, and top with ¼ teaspoon of kosher salt, ¼ teaspoon of ground black pepper, ½ teaspoon of rosemary, and ½ teaspoon of parsley.

When the grill is hot, place the marinated steaks on the grill and cook for about 4 minutes on each side for a medium steak, or until desired doneness is reached. When you turn the steaks, place the asparagus on the grill together with the potatoes on their bed of aluminum foil.

Serve each steak with half of the grilled asparagus and one crushed potato.

CHICKEN STIR-FRY

Serves 2

½ cup brown rice

1½ cups water

2 teaspoons olive oil, divided

12 ounces boneless, skinless chicken breast, cut into 1-inch strips

1 teaspoon grated ginger root

1 teaspoon chopped garlic

½ cup chopped celery

½ cup chopped carrots

½ cup chopped leeks

4 stalks scallion, chopped

¾ cup mung-bean sprouts

¼ cup lightly salted peanuts

½ cup peas

2 tablespoons low-sodium soy sauce

1 teaspoon ground black pepper

In a small pot, combine the brown rice and water. Cook covered, over low heat, for 25 minutes or until tender and all the water has been absorbed. Fluff with a fork and reserve.

In a skillet, add 1 teaspoon of olive oil and heat over medium heat. Add the chicken and sauté for 4 minutes, or until the chicken is just cooked through. Remove from the pan and reserve.

To the pan add the remaining 1 teaspoon of olive oil, the ginger root, and the garlic. Sauté for 2 minutes or until the mixture becomes slightly browned and very aromatic. Add the celery, carrots, and leeks. Sauté for 6 minutes or until softened.

When the vegetables have softened, add the scallion and mung-bean sprouts, and sauté for 2 minutes. Add the peanuts, peas, reserved chicken, soy sauce, and ground black pepper. Stir well to combine evenly, and cook about 3 minutes or until the chicken is hot.

Divide the brown rice evenly among two bowls, and top with the stir-fried chicken and the sauce from the pan.

SPICE-RUBBED TUNA
WITH **BARLEY PILAF** AND **PINEAPPLE SALSA**

Serves 2

1 cup low-sodium chicken broth or water

²/₃ cup pearl barley

1½ teaspoons kosher salt, divided

1½ teaspoons ground black pepper, divided

1 teaspoon dried oregano

1 teaspoon dried thyme

1 teaspoon cumin

1 teaspoon ground ginger

½ teaspoon ground cloves

1 cup chopped pineapple

½ small red onion, chopped

½ small red bell pepper, chopped

4 sprigs cilantro, chopped

1 tablespoon red wine vinegar

2 6-ounce tuna steaks

1 teaspoon olive oil

In a small pot, bring the chicken stock or water to a boil. When it reaches a boil, add the barley, ½ teaspoon of kosher salt, and ½ teaspoon of ground black pepper. Lower heat and simmer, covered, for 45 minutes or until the barley is soft and tender. Fluff with a fork and reserve.

To make the spice rub, in a bowl, combine the oregano, thyme, cumin, ginger, cloves, 1 teaspoon of kosher salt, and 1 teaspoon of ground black pepper. Mix to combine all ingredients.

In a mixing bowl, combine the pineapple, red onion, red pepper, cilantro, and red wine vinegar. Mix well and reserve.

Rub each tuna steak all over with 2 teaspoons of spice rub. In a skillet, heat the olive oil over medium heat. When it begins to smoke slightly, add the tuna steaks and cook 2 minutes on each side for medium rare, or until desired doneness is reached.

Divide the barley pilaf evenly among two plates. Top each serving of barley with one tuna steak and half of the pineapple salsa.

Dessert

GREEN TEA GRANITA WITH FRESH BLUEBERRIES

Serves 2

1½ cups brewed green tea, sweetened with nonnutritive sweetener to your liking
1 cup fresh blueberries

Place brewed green tea in a shallow glass baking dish, and place in the freezer. Every hour, go to the freezer and scrape the top with a fork. Allow to freeze for at least 4 hours.

Divide the granita evenly among two bowls, and top each with ½ cup of blueberries.

YOGURT MIXER WITH CHERRIES AND DARK CHOCOLATE CHIPS

Serves 1

6 ounces fat-free vanilla yogurt
¼ cup cherries, pitted
1 teaspoon dark-chocolate chips

In a blender, combine the yogurt and cherries, and blend until smooth. Mix in the chocolate chips.

GRILLED PINEAPPLE TOPPED
WITH LOW-FAT FROZEN YOGURT

Serves 4

½ medium pineapple, peeled, cored, and cut into quarters
8 ounces fat-free frozen yogurt

Preheat your grill to 350 degrees Fahrenheit. When the grill is hot, spray it with canola pan spray to prevent the pineapple from sticking.

Place the pineapple quarters on the grill and cook for 3 minutes on each side. Remove from the grill and allow to cool slightly. Top with 2 ounces of your favorite low-fat frozen yogurt.

SPICE BAKED APPLE STUFFED
WITH PRUNES AND WALNUTS

Serves 2

1 teaspoon cinnamon
½ teaspoon ground cloves
¼ teaspoon ground nutmeg
2 medium apples, whole, cored, with skin left on
2 prunes, chopped
2 tablespoons chopped walnuts
¼ cup water

Preheat oven to 350 degrees Fahrenheit. In a small bowl, combine the cinnamon, cloves, and nutmeg. Sprinkle all over and inside the cored apples. In the same bowl, combine the chopped prunes and walnuts. Stuff the prune-and-walnut mixture into the center of the cored apple.

Place the stuffed apples in a baking dish. Pour water on the bottom of the baking dish and cover with aluminum foil. Bake, covered, for 25 minutes or until the apples are soft and tender but still hold their shape.

SUPER BODY, SUPER BRAIN HEALTH TRACKING LEVEL NUMBER

Health Tracking	Week 1	Week 2	Week 3	Week 4
Weight				
BMI				
Waist-Hip Ratio*				
Resting Heart Rate				
Blood Pressure				

*Pick a measuring tape to check the waist and hip measurements. First measure your hip circumference at its widest part. Then measure your waist circumference at the belly button. People with more weight around the waist face many more health risks than people who carry more weight around their hips. Make sure the ratio keeps improving throughout time.

SUPER BODY, SUPER BRAIN
MONTHLY CALENDAR WEIGHT LOSS

Monday	Tuesday	Wednesday	Thursday	Friday	Saturday	Sunday
Day 1	Day 2	Day 3	Day 4	⬢ Day 5	Day 6	Day 7
Day 8	Day 9	Day 10	Day 11	⬢ Day 12	Day 13	Day 14
Day 15	Day 16	Day 17	Day 18	⬢ Day 19	Day 20	Day 21
Day 22	Day 23	Day 24	Day 25	⬢ Day 26	Day 27	Day 28
Day 29	Day 30	Day 31		⬢ Weight Data		

SUPER BODY, SUPER BRAIN
EXERCISE WEEKLY SCHEDULE

	Monday	Tuesday	Wednesday	Thursday	Friday	Saturday	Sunday
AM							
PM							

SUPER BODY, SUPER BRAIN
FOOD JOURNAL WEEKLY SCHEDULE

	Monday	Tuesday	Wednesday	Thursday	Friday	Saturday	Sunday
AM							
PM							
Approx. Calories							

Bibliography

Boschmann, Michael, et al. "Water-induced thermogenesis." *Journal of Clinical Endocrinology & Metabolism* 88, no. 12 (2003): 6015–6019.

Cooper Institute. "The DREW (Dose Response to Exercise) study." Dallas, 2001–2006. http://www.cooperinstitute.org/research/past/drew.cfm.

Dahl-Petersen, I., L. Eriksen, S.B. Haugaard, and F. Dela. "Physical exercise and type 2 diabetes: Is 3x10 minutes a day better than 30 minutes?" *Diabetologia* 50, no. 11 (Nov. 2007): 2245–2253.

De Matos, M.G., L. Calmeiro, and D. Da Fonseca. "Effect of physical activity on anxiety and depression." *Presse Medicale* 38, no. 5 (May 2009): 734–739.

Gates, Chee. "The workout that does it all." *O Magazine,* March 2006.

Gómez-Pinilla, F. "Brain foods: The effects of nutrients on brain function." *Nature Reviews Neuroscience* 9, no. 7 (2008): 568–578.

Greenough, W.T., and A.M. Sirevaag. "Plasticity of GFAP-immunoreactive astrocyte size and number in visual cortex of rats reared in complex environments." *Brain Research* 540, nos. 1–2 (Feb. 1, 1991): 273–278.

Hillman C.H., K.I. Erickson, and A.F. Kramer. "Be smart, exercise your heart: Exercise effects on brain and cognition." *Nature Reviews Neuroscience* 9, no. 1 (Jan. 2008): 58–65.

Jen, C.J., and H.-I. Chen. "Differential effects of treadmill running and wheel running on spatial or aversive learning and memory: Roles of amygdalar brain-derived neurotrophic factor and synaptotagmin." *Journal of Physiology* 587 (July 1, 2009): 3221–3231.

Kandel, Eric. "The molecular biology of memory storage: A dialog between genes and synapses." Nobel Lecture 21. http://nobelprize.org/nobel_prizes/medicine/laureates/2000/kandel-lecture.html.

——."Mapping Memory in the Brain." Holiday Lecture on Science, Howard Hughes Medical Institute, December 2008.

Krammer, Arthur F., et al. "Aerobic fitness is associated with hippocampal volume in elderly humans." *Hippocampus* 19, no. 10 (Oct. 2009): 1030–1039.

Leiner, H.C., A.L. Leiner, and R.S. Dow. "Cognitive and language functions of the human cerebellum." *Trends Neuroscience* 16, no. 11 (1993): 444–447.

Leiner, Henrietta C., and Alan L. Leiner. "The treasure at the bottom of the brain." http://www.newhorizons.org/neuro/leiner.htm.

Liebowitz, Michael R. *The Chemistry of Love.* New York: Penguin, 1984.

Martin, John H. *Neuroanatomy: Text and Atlas.* 3rd ed. New York: McGraw-Hill Medical, 2003.

Mayo Clinic staff. "Aerobic exercise: Top 10 reasons to get physical." http://www.mayoclinic .com/health/aerobic-exercise/EP00002.

———. "Depression and anxiety: Exercise eases symptoms." http://www.mayoclinic.com/health/ depression-and-exercise/MH00043.

Osika, Walter, and Scott M. Montgomery. "Physical control and coordination in childhood and adult obesity: Longitudinal birth cohort study." *British Medicine Journal* 337 (2008): a699.

"Physical activity and public health." *Journal of American Medical Association* 273, no. 5 (Feb. 1, 1995): 402–407.

"Physical fitness improves spatial memory, increases size of brain structure." *Science Daily,* Mar. 3, 2009.

Ponti, G., B. Peretto, and L. Bonfanti. "Genesis of neuronal and glial progenitors in the cerebellar cortex of peripuberal and adult rabbits." *PLoS ONE* 3, no. 6 (2008): e2366. http:// www.plosone.org/article/info%3Adoi%2F10.137%2Fjournal.pone.0002366.

Priya, Mohanti, et al. "Leucocytes glucose challenge stimulates reactive oxygen species (ROS) generation by leucocytes." *Journal of Clinical Endocrinology and Metabolism* 85 (2000): 2970–2973.

Ratey, John. *A User's Guide to the Brain.* New York: Vintage Books, 2002.

Sheff, David, "Whatever happened to Jane Fonda in tights?" *New York Times,* Feb. 8, 2007.

Small, Scott A., and Fred H. Gage, et al. "An in vivo correlate of exercise-induced neurogenesis in the adult dentate gyrus." Proceedings of the National Academy of Sciences of United States of America, vol. 104, no. 13 (March 27, 2007): 5638–5643. http://www.pnas.org/content/104/13/5638.

Stanford University. "Training effects of long versus short bouts of exercise in healthy subjects." *American Journal of Cardiology* 65 (1990): 1010–1013.

Van Praag, Henriette, Tiffany Shubert, Chunmei Zhao, and Fred H. Gage. "Exercise enhances learning and hippocampal neurogenesis in aged mice "*Journal of Neuroscience* (2005): 8680–8685.

Yamori, Y., International Center for Research on Primary Prevention of Cardiovascular Diseases, et al. "Worldwide epidemic of obesity: Hope for Japanese diets." *Clinical Experimental Pharmacology and Physiology* 31, suppl. 2 (Dec. 2004): S2–S4.

Other Sources

American Heart Association. http://www.americanheart.org.

American Diabetes Association. http://www.diabetes.org.

U.S. Surgeon General Report, 2008. http://www.surgeongeneral.gov.

Acknowledgments

I never thought I would be writing this page and am thrilled that my incredible six-year journey—my "impossible dream"—has become a reality. I would like to thank so many people, starting with my literary agent, Eileen Cope of Trident Media, who believed in me without hesitation, and the spectacular writer Karen Moline, who helped me put into words all of my excitement and passion for this program. Thanks to my publisher, Harper-One, especially Mark Tauber and my dearest editor Nancy Hancock. Nancy has been so supportive, and has made terrific suggestions all along the way. I have been lucky to work with such a superb and phenomenal team at HarperOne.

This book would never have been possible without the help of all my clients, who have taught me so much about the brain and the body. In particular, I want to thank Amy Gross, who has helped me with wise advice, direction, and encouragement; Ellen, Dick, and Jill Seelig for their constant guidance; and Lori Oshansky for her intense involvement. In addition, greatly appreciated are my best clients, including Amiee Telsey, Richard Friesner, Marty Fleischer, Andrea Bierstein, Susan and Tucker York, Wendy Belzberg, Gaylord Nelly, Indran Purusothaman, Agnes Czarnik, and Ilaria Bulgari.

A very special thanks to the readers of O, The Oprah Magazine for sending me hundreds of emails and letters encouraging me to write this book.

Special thanks to neurobiologist John Martin, Ph.D., who encouraged me to take my program to the next level and offered me invaluable information about how the brain relates to movement. Neurologist Lice Ghilardi, M.D., spent several hours explaining to me how the brain and the body interact and the importance of specific physical movements. Gregory Lombardo, M.D., taught me invaluable lessons about the human mind. I am so grateful to you all for helping to make my program a better one.

My sincere thanks to the entire panel of experts I consulted and interviewed for this book especially John Martin, Ph.D.; Lice Ghilardi. M.D.; Michael Liebowitz. M.D.; Charles Hillman, Ph.D.; Alvaro Fernandez; Wendy Suzuki, Ph.D.; Bradley Radwaner, M.D.; Professor Luca Bonfanti. Ph.D.; Bente Klarlund Pedersen, M.D.; Terrance Capistrant, M.D.; Nelly Szlachter, M.D.; Patrick Cohn, Ph.D.; and Arthur Krammer, Ph.D.

Special thanks go to Sharon Salzberg and Rebecca Victor-Hobert for their help.

Also, special thanks to a remarkable nutritionist, Olinka Podany, M.S., R.D., who contributed to the nutrition section. Thanks also to Recipe Consultants for preparing the unique recipes that I've included, especially Anthony Marzuillo for his guidance.

I am truly indebted to my close friends for their generosity of spirit and their listening ears throughout this journey. I am so thankful to Jessica Williams, Elias Plagianos, Rick Aguilar, Gaby Baltis, Maria Dorfner, Chee Gates, Sonsoles , Miguel Angel Medina, Ben Golburg, Laura Corby, Rachel Crump, Carlos Saavedra, Ana Prieto, Santiago Mora, Ivona kak, the Clauson family, and many more.

I am deeply grateful to the governor of Minnesota, Tim Pawlenty, and the mayor of St. Paul, Christopher Coleman, who awarded me the Fitness Excellence Award and encouraged me to write this book.

Thanks especially to a public school in the Bronx, PS 277, especially Principal Cheryl Tyler and gym teacher Euridice Johnson. And thanks to Englewood Hospital for their interest.

I have had the great fortune to study at and work with Ramiro de Maeztu High School, the Estudiantes basketball team in Madrid, Autónoma University, the New York Sports Club, and the National Academy of Sports Medicine. Thank you to the students, professors, teammates, and professionals I have met for the invaluable lessons you've taught me.

Thanks to all my Facebook fans and friends, who have been extremely enthusiastic about my program.

I've saved these last lines for my absolute pillar, and my secret weapon: my family. I am sure that I would never have made it so far without their constant support and encouragement. My special thanks to my parents, Pedro and Lee, and my siblings, John and Diana, who listened to endless conversations during this book's journey. I know they were a little nervous when I made the leap from investment banking to fitness, but like they've taught me, find your inner passion and make it your most valuable asset. Thanks to my dear godfather, Miguel, and Julia Sanchez for their constant encouragement. And many more and you know you are out there.

About the Author

Michael Gonzalez-Wallace has been involved in athletic sports for over twenty years. Michael's athletic career includes many years of playing semiprofessional basketball in Spain, where his team, Estudiantes Madrid, won the Spanish National Competition (similar to the NCAA in the United States) and where he was named the MVP of the final, in May 1993. In 1995 the Spanish basketball federation certified Michael as a strength trainer and basketball coach, providing him the opportunity to develop his teaching skills. In his more than fifteen years of involvement with basketball, Michael learned the important concepts of teamwork, leadership, muscle coordination, and physical strength training. As a student at the Universidad Autónoma de Madrid (a top Spanish economics school), he added the art of doing research to his skill set. In 2002 he become a personal trainer for the New York Sports Clubs group and received a certification from the National Academy of Sports Medicine. He has been featured in *Redbook; Prevention; O, The Oprah Magazine;* and *Fitness* magazines and on msnbc.com and CNN. He lives in New York City.